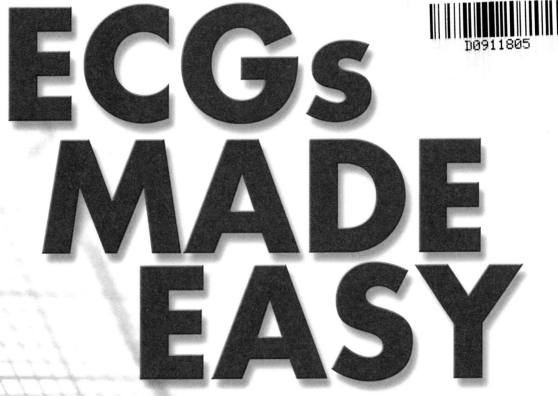

ECGs MADE EASY
Study Cards

Barbara Aehlert, RN

Southwest EMS Education, Inc.
Phoenix, Arizona

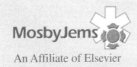

MosbyJems

An Affiliate of Elsevier

D0911805

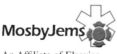

MosbyJems

An Affiliate of Elsevier

11830 Westline Industrial Drive
St. Louis, Missouri 63146

ECGs MADE EASY STUDY CARDS   ISBN   0-323-02311-8
Copyright © 2004, Mosby, Inc. All rights reserved.

NOTICE

Cardiography is an ever-changing field. Standard safety precautions must be followed, but as new research and clinical experience broaden our knowledge, changes in treatment and drug therapy may become necessary or appropriate. Readers are advised to check the most current product information provided by the manufacturer of each drug to be administered to verify the recommended dose, the method and duration of administration, and contraindications. It is the responsibility of the licensed health care provider, relying on experience and knowledge of the patient, to determine dosages and the best treatment for each individual patient. Neither the publisher nor the author assumes any liability for any injury and/or damage to persons or property arising from this publication.

International Standard Book Number 0-323-02311-8

Acquisitions Editor: Linda Honeycutt
Developmental Editor: Laura Bayless
Project Manager: Peggy Fagen
Designer: Bill Drone

Printed in the United States

Last digit is the print number: 9   8   7   6   5   4   3   2   1

NOTE TO THE READER

- These ECG cards are designed to assist you in mastering ECG interpretation. The first 25 cards, in green, review cardiac anatomy and physiology and electrophysiology. The last 50 cards, in blue, focus on 12-lead ECG review. The remainder of the cards, in red, have been placed in random order and offer a review of 3-lead ECGs.

- Determination of heart rate on these ECG cards will require calculations using the large box or small box method. Use of an ECG ruler will result in **inaccurate** results because the rhythm strips have been reduced in size.

- These cards have been perforated for easy removal from the book. You are encouraged to pull out the cards you feel you need more practice with. Link them together through the prepunched holes to form your own custom card decks for quick review.

ABOUT THE AUTHOR

Barbara Aehlert, R.N., is the President/CEO of Southwest EMS Education, Inc., in Phoenix, Arizona. She has been a registered nurse for more than 20 years with clinical experience in medical/surgical and critical care nursing and, for the past 15 years, in prehospital education. As an active instructor, Barbara regularly teaches courses related to the care of the adult cardiac patient and takes a special interest in teaching basic dysrhythmia recognition to nurses and paramedics.

CONTENTS

- Label the following coronary arteries:
  - Circumflex
  - Posterior descending
  - Anterior descending
  - Marginal
  - Right coronary artery
  - Left main coronary artery

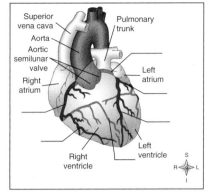

Superior vena cava · Pulmonary trunk · Aorta · Aortic semilunar valve · Right atrium · Left atrium · Left ventricle · Right ventricle · S R L I

- Name the ECG waveform that represents atrial depolarization.
- Name the ECG waveform that represents ventricular depolarization.

- What is meant by the term "atrial kick"?

- What does the ST-segment represent on the ECG?
- What does the T wave represent on the ECG?

- Name the two types of cardiac cells and describe their function.

- Explain the significance of each of the numbers illustrated below and their relationship to ventricular depolarization or repolarization.

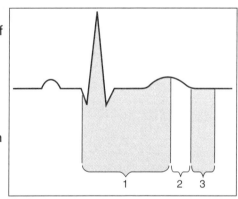

1   2   3

Depolarization and repolarization are changes that occur in the heart when an impulse forms and spreads throughout the myocardium. These changes occur because of the movement of ions across the cell membrane.

- Do these illustrations reflect depolarization or repolarization?

Na⁺ Na⁺ Na⁺ Na⁺ Na⁺

Locate the following parts of the conduction system on this illustration:
- Right bundle branch
- Left bundle branch
- AV node
- SA node
- Purkinje fibers
- Bundle of His

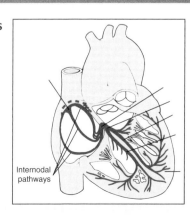

Internodal pathways

On the ECG:
- The *P wave* represents atrial depolarization.
- The *QRS complex* represents ventricular depolarization.

- Coronary arteries and heart valves

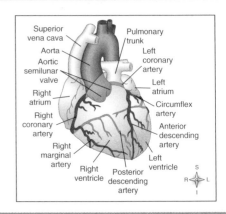

- The ST-segment represents early ventricular repolarization.
- The T wave presents ventricular repolarization.

- During ventricular relaxation (diastole), the ventricles fill passively with approximately 70% of the blood that has accumulated in the atria.
- Contraction of the atria forces the remaining atrial blood into the ventricles.
- This contribution accounts for 10% to 30% of the cardiac output and is called *atrial kick.*
- Because atrial kick can account for up to 30% of the patient's cardiac output, a loss of atrial kick (as in dysrhythmias such as atrial fibrillation) may result in serious signs and symptoms.

1. Absolute refractory period
   - Onset of QRS complex to approximately peak of T wave
   - Cardiac cells cannot be stimulated to conduct an electrical impulse, no matter how strong the stimulus
2. Relative refractory period
   - Corresponds with the downslope of the T wave
   - Cardiac cells can be stimulated to depolarize if the stimulus is strong enough
3. Supernormal period
   - Corresponds with the end of the T wave
   - A weaker than normal stimulus can cause depolarization of cardiac cells

- Myocardial (working) cells (also known as mechanical cells) are found in the myocardium. These cells contain contractile filaments. When electrically stimulated, these filaments slide together and the myocardial cell contracts.
- Electrical (pacemaker) cells are found in the electrical conduction system. They are responsible for the spontaneous generation and conduction of electrical impulses.

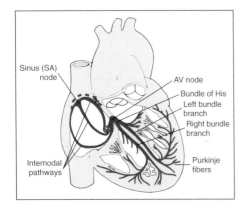

- These illustrations reflect depolarization.
- When the cardiac muscle cell is stimulated, the cell is said to depolarize. The inside of the cell becomes more positive because of the entry of sodium (Na^+) ions into the cell through Na^+ membrane channels. Thus depolarization occurs because of the inward diffusion of Na^+.

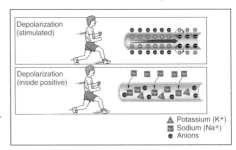

- The position of the positive electrode on the body determines the portion of the heart "seen" by each lead. Each lead senses the magnitude and direction of the electrical forces caused by the spread of waves of depolarization and repolarization throughout the heart.
- Look at this illustration and (for each lead) determine if the ECG waveform will be biphasic, positive, or negative.

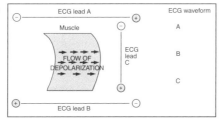

- Name the lead illustrated here.

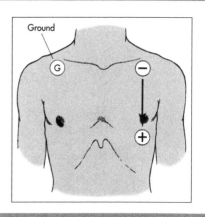

- Name the lead illustrated here.

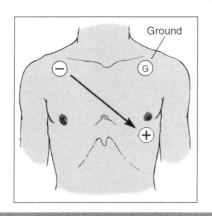

Label the following on this illustration:
- Voltage (amplitude) axis
- Time axis
- P wave, Q wave, R wave, S wave, T wave
- PR interval and its normal value
- QRS duration and its normal value
- ST-segment
- QT interval and its normal value

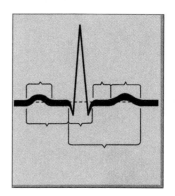

- Do these illustrations reflect depolarization or repolarization?

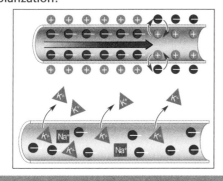

- Label precordial leads V_1, V_2, V_3, V_4, V_5, and V_6 on this illustration.

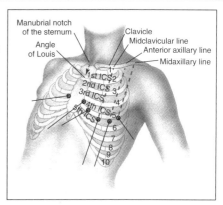

Label the following on this illustration:
- Voltage (amplitude) axis
- Time axis
- P wave, Q wave, R wave, S wave, T wave
- Atrial depolarization
- Ventricular depolarization
- Ventricular repolarization

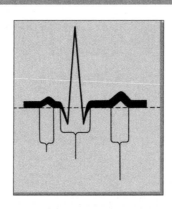

- Name the lead illustrated here.

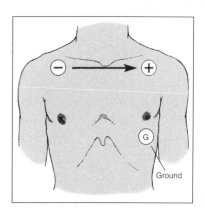

- Lead III.
- Lead III records the difference in electrical potential between the left leg (+) and left arm (−) electrodes. The positive electrode is placed below the left pectoral muscle (or on the left leg), and the negative electrode is placed just below the left clavicle (or on the left arm). The third electrode is a ground that minimizes electrical activity from other sources.

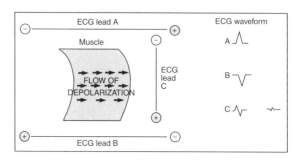

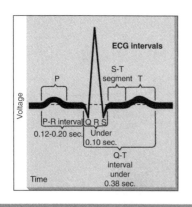

- Lead II.
- Lead II records the difference in electrical potential between the left leg (+) and right arm (−) electrodes. The positive electrode is placed below the left pectoral muscle (or on the left leg), and the negative electrode is placed just below the right clavicle (or on the right arm). The third electrode is a ground that minimizes electrical activity from other sources.

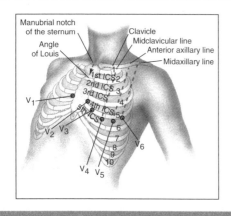

- These illustrations reflect repolarization.
- After the cell depolarizes, the diffusion of Na^+ into the cell stops. Potassium (K^+) is allowed to diffuse out of the cell, leaving the anions (negatively charged ions) inside the cell. Thus repolarization occurs because of the outward diffusion of K^+.

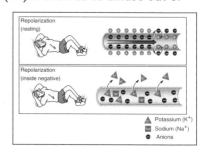

- Lead I.
- Lead I records the difference in electrical potential between the left arm (+) and right arm (−) electrodes. The positive electrode is placed just below the left clavicle (or on the left arm), and the negative electrode is placed just below the right clavicle (or on the right arm). The third electrode is a ground that minimizes electrical activity from other sources.

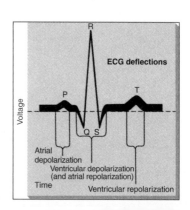

◆ One method used to calculate heart rate requires determining the number of large boxes between two consecutive R waves (ventricular rate) or P waves (atrial rate).

◆ Complete the following table.

NO. OF LARGE BOXES	HEART RATE (BEATS/MIN)	NO. OF LARGE BOXES	HEART RATE (BEATS/MIN)
1		6	
2		7	
3		8	
4		9	
5		10	

◆ Complete the following table regarding standard limb leads.

LEAD	POSITIVE ELECTRODE POSITION	NEGATIVE ELECTRODE POSITION	HEART SURFACE VIEWED
I			
II			
III			

◆ Distortion of an ECG tracing by electrical activity that is noncardiac in origin is called artifact. What is the most likely cause of artifact in this ECG strip?

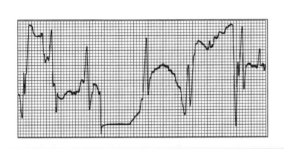

◆ Complete the following table regarding the augmented limb leads.

LEAD	POSITIVE ELECTRODE POSITION	HEART SURFACE VIEWED
aVR		
aVL		
aVF		

◆ A QRS-complex may appear in various forms. Label each waveform in this illustration.

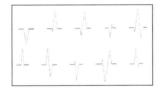

◆ Complete the following table regarding the precordial leads.

LEAD	POSITIVE ELECTRODE POSITION	HEART SURFACE VIEWED
V_1		
V_2		
V_3		
V_4		
V_5		
V_6		

◆ What is the most likely cause of artifact in this ECG strip?

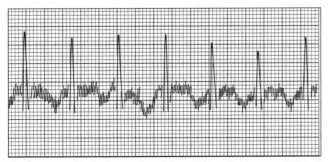

◆ What is the most likely cause of artifact in this ECG strip?

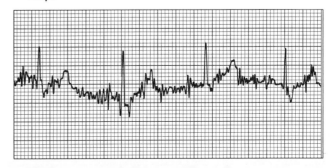

LEAD	POSITIVE ELECTRODE POSITION	NEGATIVE ELECTRODE POSITION	HEART SURFACE VIEWED
I	Left arm	Right arm	Lateral
II	Left leg	Right arm	Inferior
III	Left leg	Left arm	Inferior

NO. OF LARGE BOXES	HEART RATE (BEATS/MIN)	NO. OF LARGE BOXES	HEART RATE (BEATS/MIN)
1	300	6	50
2	150	7	43
3	100	8	38
4	75	9	33
5	60	10	30

LEAD	POSITIVE ELECTRODE POSITION	HEART SURFACE VIEWED
aVR	Right arm	None
aVL	Left arm	Lateral
aVF	Left leg	Inferior

◆ An irregular baseline may be identified by bizarre, irregular deflections of the baseline on the ECG paper. This may be the result of a broken lead wire, poor electrical contact, or a loose electrode.

LEAD	POSITIVE ELECTRODE POSITION	HEART SURFACE VIEWED
V₁	Right side of sternum, fourth intercostal space	Septum
V₂	Left side of sternum, 4th intercostal space	Septum
V₃	Midway between V₂ and V₄	Anterior
V₄	Left midclavicular line, fifth intercostal space	Anterior
V₅	Left anterior axillary line at same level as V₄	Lateral
V₆	Left midaxillary line at same level as V₄	Lateral

A Q wave is the first negative deflection following the P wave. The first positive deflection in the QRS complex is called an R wave. A negative deflection following the R wave is called an S wave. Not every QRS-complex contains a Q wave, R wave, and S wave.

If the QRS complex consists entirely of a positive waveform, it is called an R wave. If the complex consists entirely of a negative waveform, it is called a QS wave. If there are two positive deflections in the same complex, the second is called R prime and is written R'. If there are two negative deflections following an R wave, the second is written S'.

Capital (uppercase) letters designate waveforms of relatively large amplitude and small (lowercase) letters are used to label relatively small waveforms.

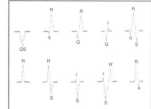

◆ A wandering baseline may occur because of normal respiratory movement (particularly when electrodes have been applied directly over the ribs) or because of poor electrode contact with the patient's skin. Seizures, shivering, tense muscles, or Parkinson's disease may cause muscle tremor artifact. Consider clipping the ECG cable to the patient's clothing to minimize excessive movement.

◆ 60-cycle interference. This may be caused by improperly grounded electrical equipment or other electrical interference.
◆ If 60-cycle interference is observed, check for crossing of the cable wires with other electrical wires (e.g., bed control) and frayed or broken wires. Verify that all electrical equipment is properly grounded and that the cable electrode connections are clean.

◆ Indicate the intrinsic rate for each of the following pacemaker sites:
  ◆ Sinoatrial (SA) node: _____
  ◆ Atrioventricular (AV) junction: _____
  ◆ Purkinje fibers: _____

◆ SA node: <u>60 to 100 beats/min</u>
◆ AV junction: <u>40 to 60 beats/min</u>
◆ Purkinje fibers: <u>20 to 40 beats/min</u>

RHYTHM IDENTIFICATION

- This rhythm strip is from a 35-year-old woman complaining of chest pain and palpitations. Identify the rhythm (lead II).

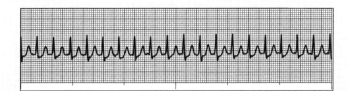

RHYTHM IDENTIFICATION

- This rhythm strip is from a 33-year-old woman complaining of abdominal pain. Identify the rhythm (lead II).

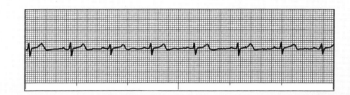

RHYTHM IDENTIFICATION

- This rhythm strip is from a 69-year-old woman complaining of shortness of breath. She has a history of chronic obstructive pulmonary disease. Identify the rhythm.

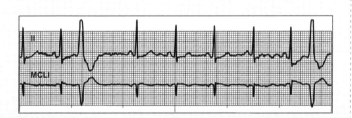

RHYTHM IDENTIFICATION

- This rhythm strip is from a 57-year-old man with no cardiac history. Identify the rhythm (lead II).

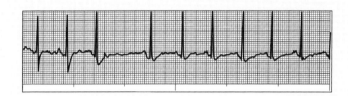

RHYTHM IDENTIFICATION

- This rhythm strip is from a 96-year-old man complaining of chest pain and palpitations. Medications include Lanoxin and Coumadin. Identify the rhythm.

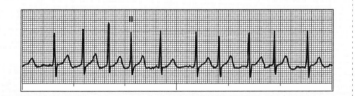

RHYTHM IDENTIFICATION

- Identify the rhythm (lead II).

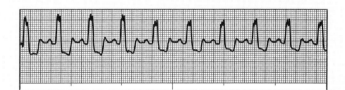

RHYTHM IDENTIFICATION

- This rhythm strip is from an 8-month-old infant after a seizure. Identify the rhythm (lead I).

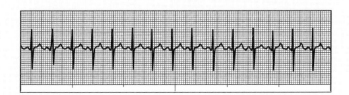

RHYTHM IDENTIFICATION

- This rhythm strip is from a 75-year-old man complaining of chest pain that has been present for 20 minutes. He rates his pain an 8 on a 1 to 10 scale. His blood pressure is 172/98. Identify the rhythm (lead II).

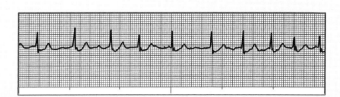

RHYTHM IDENTIFICATION

Sinus rhythm
- ◆ Ventricular rhythm   Regular
- ◆ Ventricular rate   71/min
- ◆ Atrial rhythm   Regular
- ◆ Atrial rate   71/min
- ◆ PRI: 0.12 second
- ◆ QRS: 0.08 second

RHYTHM IDENTIFICATION

Narrow QRS tachycardia (SVT) with ST-segment depression
- ◆ Ventricular rhythm   Regular
- ◆ Ventricular rate   188/min
- ◆ Atrial rhythm   Unable to determine
- ◆ Atrial rate   Unable to determine
- ◆ PRI: Unable to determine
- ◆ QRS: 0.06 second

RHYTHM IDENTIFICATION

Sinus rhythm with a nonconducted PAC
- ◆ Ventricular rhythm   Irregular
- ◆ Ventricular rate   57 to 100/min
- ◆ Atrial rhythm   Irregular
- ◆ Atrial rate   75 to 167/min
- ◆ PRI: 0.18 second
- ◆ QRS: 0.08 second

RHYTHM IDENTIFICATION

Sinus rhythm with uniform PVCs
- ◆ Ventricular rhythm   Regular except for the events
- ◆ Ventricular rate   80/min (sinus beats)
- ◆ Atrial rhythm   Regular except for the events
- ◆ Atrial rate   80/min (sinus beats)
- ◆ PRI: 0.12 to 0.14 second (sinus beats)
- ◆ QRS: 0.06 second (sinus beats)

RHYTHM IDENTIFICATION

Sinus rhythm with a wide QRS, ST-segment depression
- ◆ Ventricular rhythm   Regular
- ◆ Ventricular rate   94/min
- ◆ Atrial rhythm   Regular
- ◆ Atrial rate   94/min
- ◆ PRI: 0.18 second
- ◆ QRS: 0.12 second (wide, probably due to right bundle branch block)

RHYTHM IDENTIFICATION

Atrial fibrillation
- ◆ Ventricular rhythm   Irregular
- ◆ Ventricular rate   88 to 130/min
- ◆ Atrial rhythm   Unable to determine
- ◆ Atrial rate   Unable to determine
- ◆ PRI: Unable to determine
- ◆ QRS: 0.08 second

RHYTHM IDENTIFICATION

Atrial fibrillation
- ◆ Ventricular rhythm   Irregular
- ◆ Ventricular rate   79 to 125/min
- ◆ Atrial rhythm   Unable to determine
- ◆ Atrial rate   Unable to determine
- ◆ PRI: Unable to determine
- ◆ QRS: 0.06 to 0.08 second

RHYTHM IDENTIFICATION

Sinus tachycardia
- ◆ Ventricular rhythm   Regular
- ◆ Ventricular rate   150/min
- ◆ Atrial rhythm   Regular
- ◆ Atrial rate   150/min
- ◆ PRI: 0.12 second
- ◆ QRS: 0.06 to 0.08 second

RHYTHM IDENTIFICATION

◆ This rhythm strip is from a 74-year-old woman with difficulty breathing. Identify the rhythm.

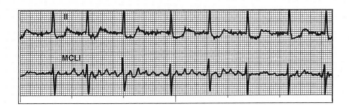

RHYTHM IDENTIFICATION

◆ This rhythm strip is from a 19-year-old man complaining of shortness of breath. Identify the rhythm (lead II).

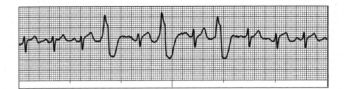

RHYTHM IDENTIFICATION

◆ This rhythm strip is from a 70-year-old man complaining of weakness. Identify the rhythm.

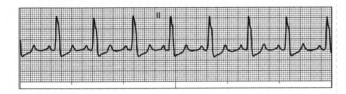

RHYTHM IDENTIFICATION

◆ This rhythm strip is from a 24-year-old woman complaining of weakness and fatigue. Identify the rhythm (lead II).

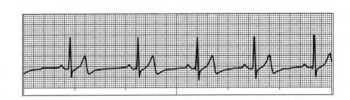

RHYTHM IDENTIFICATION

◆ This rhythm strip is from a 90-year-old woman complaining of difficulty breathing. Identify the rhythm (lead II).

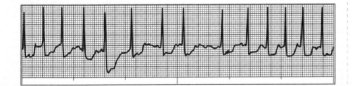

RHYTHM IDENTIFICATION

◆ This rhythm strip is from a 59-year-old woman complaining of chest pain. She has a history of congestive heart failure and seizures. Identify the rhythm (lead II).

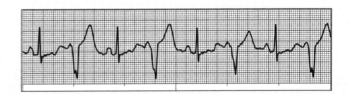

RHYTHM IDENTIFICATION

◆ This rhythm strip is from a 20-year-old woman, the victim of a tricyclic antidepressant overdose. Identify the rhythm (lead I).

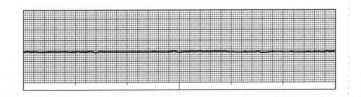

RHYTHM IDENTIFICATION

◆ These rhythm strips are from a 35-year-old man complaining his heart is racing. Blood pressure is 100/80. Identify the rhythm.

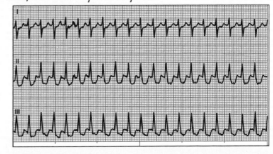

RHYTHM IDENTIFICATION

Sinus tachycardia with uniform PVCs
- Ventricular rhythm — Regular except for the event
- Ventricular rate — Approximately 110/min (sinus beats)
- Atrial rhythm — Regular except for the event
- Atrial rate — Approximately 110/min (sinus beats)
- PRI: — 0.16 second (sinus beats)
- QRS: — 0.08 second (sinus beats)

RHYTHM IDENTIFICATION

Atrial flutter
- Ventricular rhythm — Irregular
- Ventricular rate — 75 to 107/min
- Atrial rhythm — Unable to determine
- Atrial rate — Unable to determine
- PRI: — Unable to determine
- QRS: — 0.08 second

RHYTHM IDENTIFICATION

Sinus bradyarrhythmia
- Ventricular rhythm — Irregular
- Ventricular rate — 45 to 54/min
- Atrial rhythm — Irregular
- Atrial rate — 45 to 54/min
- PRI: — 0.18 second
- QRS: — 0.08 second

RHYTHM IDENTIFICATION

Sinus rhythm with a wide QRS
- Ventricular rhythm — Regular
- Ventricular rate — 71/min
- Atrial rhythm — Regular
- Atrial rate — 71/min
- PRI: — 0.16 to 0.20 second
- QRS: — 0.12 to 0.14 second

RHYTHM IDENTIFICATION

Sinus bradycardia with ventricular bigeminy
- Ventricular rhythm — Regular except for the event
- Ventricular rate — 39/min (sinus beats)
- Atrial rhythm — Regular except for the event
- Atrial rate — 39/min (sinus beats)
- PRI: — 0.20 second (sinus beats)
- QRS: — 0.08 second (sinus beats)

RHYTHM IDENTIFICATION

Atrial fibrillation (uncontrolled)
- Ventricular rhythm — Irregular
- Ventricular rate — 83 to 167/min
- Atrial rhythm — Unable to determine
- Atrial rate — Unable to determine
- PRI: — Unable to determine
- QRS: — 0.06 to 0.08 second

RHYTHM IDENTIFICATION

Narrow-QRS tachycardia (SVT)
- Ventricular rhythm — Regular
- Ventricular rate — 196/min
- Atrial rhythm — Unable to determine
- Atrial rate — Unable to determine
- PRI: — Unable to determine
- QRS: — 0.08 second

RHYTHM IDENTIFICATION

P-wave asystole
- Ventricular rhythm — None
- Ventricular rate — None
- Atrial rhythm — Regular
- Atrial rate — Approximately 38/min
- PRI: — None
- QRS: — None

RHYTHM IDENTIFICATION

◆ Identify the rhythm (lead II).

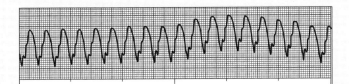

RHYTHM IDENTIFICATION

◆ Identify the rhythm (lead II).

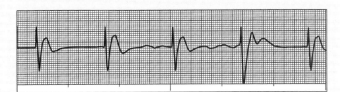

RHYTHM IDENTIFICATION

◆ These rhythm strips are from a 63-year-old man complaining of epigastric pain. Identify the rhythm.

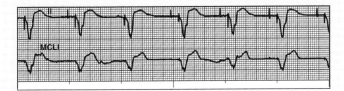

RHYTHM IDENTIFICATION

◆ This rhythm strip is from a 78-year-old woman with an altered level of responsiveness. She quickly became unresponsive, apneic, and pulseless. Identify the rhythm (lead II).

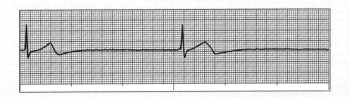

RHYTHM IDENTIFICATION

◆ This rhythm strip is from a 70-year-old man who sustained second-degree burns over 20% of his body. He has a history of diabetes, coronary artery disease, and hypertension. Blood pressure is 150/79. Respirations are 13. Identify the rhythm (lead II).

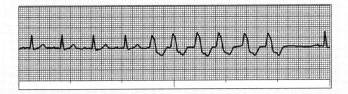

RHYTHM IDENTIFICATION

◆ This rhythm strip is from a 71-year-old man complaining of shoulder pain that has been present for 3 weeks. Identify the rhythm (lead II).

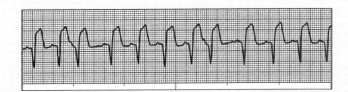

RHYTHM IDENTIFICATION

◆ This rhythm strip is from an 83-year-old woman with syncope. Identify the rhythm (lead II).

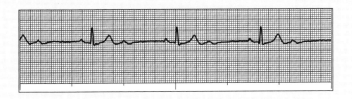

RHYTHM IDENTIFICATION

◆ Identify the rhythm (lead II).

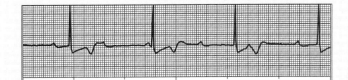

RHYTHM IDENTIFICATION

Accelerated idioventricular rhythm (AIVR)
- Ventricular rhythm — Regular
- Ventricular rate — 45/min
- Atrial rhythm — None
- Atrial rate — None
- PRI: — None
- QRS: — 0.12 second

RHYTHM IDENTIFICATION

Monomorphic ventricular tachycardia (VT)
- Ventricular rhythm — Regular
- Ventricular rate — 188/min
- Atrial rhythm — Unable to determine
- Atrial rate — Unable to determine
- PRI: — Unable to determine
- QRS: — 0.18 second

RHYTHM IDENTIFICATION

Junctional bradycardia
- Ventricular rhythm — Regular
- Ventricular rate — 23/min
- Atrial rhythm — None
- Atrial rate — None
- PRI: — None
- QRS: — 0.08 to 0.12 second

Note: The rhythm that followed this rhythm strip was asystole.

RHYTHM IDENTIFICATION

100% paced rhythm—AV sequential pacemaker
- Atrial paced activity? — Yes
- Ventricular paced activity? — Yes
- Paced interval rate? — 88

RHYTHM IDENTIFICATION

Sinus tachycardia with PACs and ST-segment elevation
- Ventricular rhythm — Regular except for the events
- Ventricular rate — 115/min (sinus beats)
- Atrial rhythm — Regular except for the events
- Atrial rate — 115/min (sinus beats)
- PRI: — 0.12 second (sinus beats)
- QRS: — 0.08 second (sinus beats)

RHYTHM IDENTIFICATION

Sinus rhythm with a run of ventricular tachycardia
- Ventricular rhythm — Regular except for the event
- Ventricular rate — 96/min (sinus beats)
- Atrial rhythm — Regular except for the event
- Atrial rate — 96/min (sinus beats)
- PRI: — 0.20 second (sinus beats)
- QRS: — 0.08 second (sinus beats)

RHYTHM IDENTIFICATION

Complete AV block with ST-segment depression and inverted T waves
- Ventricular rhythm — Regular
- Ventricular rate — 38/min
- Atrial rhythm — Regular
- Atrial rate — 68/min
- PRI: — Varies
- QRS: — 0.06 second

RHYTHM IDENTIFICATION

Second-degree AV block, 2:1 conduction, probably type I
- Ventricular rhythm — Regular
- Ventricular rate — 36/min
- Atrial rhythm — Regular
- Atrial rate — 72/min
- PRI: — 0.20 to 0.22 second
- QRS: — 0.06 to 0.08 second

RHYTHM IDENTIFICATION

- ◆ This rhythm strip is from a 90-year-old woman with a history of congestive heart failure. She is unresponsive and on a ventilator. Identify the rhythm (lead II).

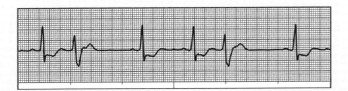

RHYTHM IDENTIFICATION

- ◆ This rhythm strip is from an 82-year-old man complaining of back pain. Identify the rhythm (top = lead II; bottom = MCL1).

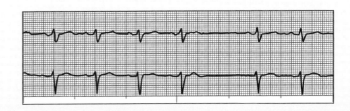

RHYTHM IDENTIFICATION

- ◆ Identify the rhythm.

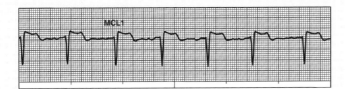

RHYTHM IDENTIFICATION

- ◆ This rhythm strip is from an 86-year-old woman who experienced a cardiopulmonary arrest. The initial rhythm was asystole. The following rhythm resulted after IV administration of epinephrine and atropine. Identify the rhythm (lead III).

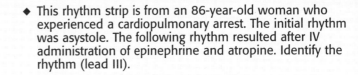

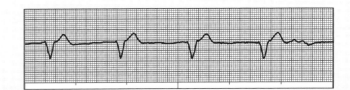

RHYTHM IDENTIFICATION

- ◆ Identify the rhythm (lead III).

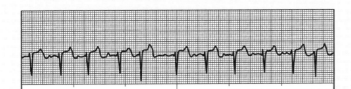

RHYTHM IDENTIFICATION

- ◆ This rhythm strip is from a 69-year-old man complaining of shortness of breath. Lung sounds reveal bilateral rales. Blood pressure 160/58. Identify the rhythm (lead II).

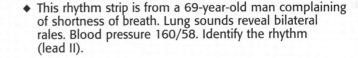

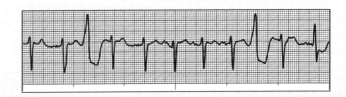

RHYTHM IDENTIFICATION

- ◆ This rhythm strip is from an 83-year-old woman with syncope. Identify the rhythm (lead II).

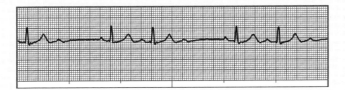

RHYTHM IDENTIFICATION

- ◆ Identify the rhythm (lead II).

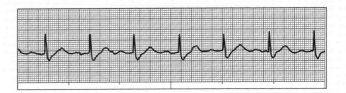

RHYTHM IDENTIFICATION

Sinus rhythm with a nonconducted PAC
- Ventricular rhythm   Irregular
- Ventricular rate   41-73/min
- Atrial rhythm   Irregular
- Atrial rate   56-125/min
- PRI: 0.20 second
- QRS: 0.12 second

RHYTHM IDENTIFICATION

Sinus rhythm with uniform PVCs, ST-segment depression, and inverted T waves
- Ventricular rhythm   Regular except for the event
- Ventricular rate   62/min (sinus beats)
- Atrial rhythm   Regular except for the event
- Atrial rate   62/min (sinus beats)
- PRI: 0.18 to 0.20 second (sinus beats)
- QRS: 0.10 second (sinus beats)

RHYTHM IDENTIFICATION

Idioventricular rhythm (also called ventricular escape rhythm)
- Ventricular rhythm   Regular
- Ventricular rate   40/min
- Atrial rhythm   None
- Atrial rate   None
- PRI: None
- QRS: 0.18 second

RHYTHM IDENTIFICATION

Sinus rhythm with first-degree AV block, ST-segment elevation
- Ventricular rhythm   Regular
- Ventricular rate   68/min
- Atrial rhythm   Regular
- Atrial rate   68/min
- PRI: 0.24 second
- QRS: 0.06 to 0.08 second

RHYTHM IDENTIFICATION

Sinus tachycardia with uniform PVCs
- Ventricular rhythm   Regular except for the events
- Ventricular rate   107/min (sinus beats)
- Atrial rhythm   Regular except for the events
- Atrial rate   107/min (sinus beats)
- PRI: 0.20 second (sinus beats)
- QRS: 0.08 second (sinus beats)

RHYTHM IDENTIFICATION

Sinus rhythm with two PJCs, ST-segment elevation
- Ventricular rhythm   Regular except for the event
- Ventricular rate   83/min (sinus beats)
- Atrial rhythm   Regular except for the event
- Atrial rate   83/min (sinus beats)
- PRI: 0.20 second
- QRS: 0.08 to 0.10 second

RHYTHM IDENTIFICATION

Sinus rhythm with first-degree AV block, ST-segment depression
- Ventricular rhythm   Regular
- Ventricular rate   68/min
- Atrial rhythm   Regular
- Atrial rate   68/min
- PRI: 0.28 second
- QRS: 0.06 second

RHYTHM IDENTIFICATION

Second-degree AV block, type I
- Ventricular rhythm   Irregular
- Ventricular rate   38 to 75/min
- Atrial rhythm   Regular
- Atrial rate   75/min
- PRI: Lengthening
- QRS: 0.06 to 0.08 second

RHYTHM IDENTIFICATION

◆ Identify the rhythm.

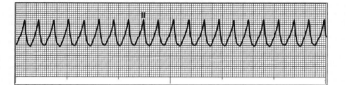

RHYTHM IDENTIFICATION

◆ Identify the rhythm (lead MCLI).

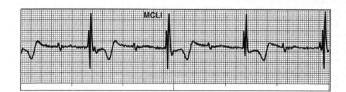

RHYTHM IDENTIFICATION

◆ Identify the rhythm (lead II).

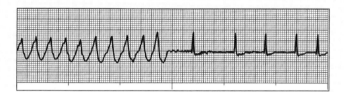

RHYTHM IDENTIFICATION

◆ This rhythm strip is from a 52-year-old man found unresponsive, apneic, and pulseless. Identify the rhythm (lead II).

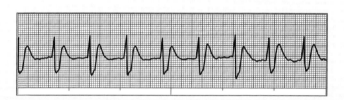

RHYTHM IDENTIFICATION

◆ Identify the rhythm (lead II).

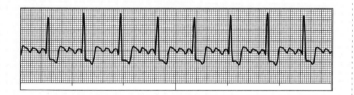

RHYTHM IDENTIFICATION

◆ Identify the rhythm (lead II).

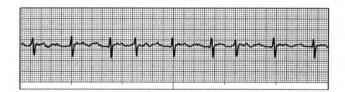

RHYTHM IDENTIFICATION

◆ Identify the rhythm (lead II).

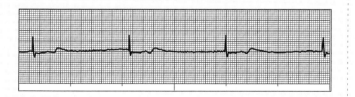

RHYTHM IDENTIFICATION

◆ Identify the rhythm (lead II).

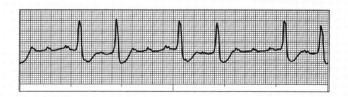

RHYTHM IDENTIFICATION

Complete (third-degree) AV block with inverted T waves
- Ventricular rhythm   Regular
- Ventricular rate   35/min
- Atrial rhythm   Regular
- Atrial rate   71/min
- PRI: Varies
- QRS: 0.12 second

RHYTHM IDENTIFICATION

Monomorphic ventricular tachycardia
- Ventricular rhythm   Regular
- Ventricular rate   214/min
- Atrial rhythm   Unable to determine
- Atrial rate   Unable to determine
- PRI: Unable to determine
- QRS: 0.14 second

RHYTHM IDENTIFICATION

Accelerated idioventricular rhythm (AIVR)
- Ventricular rhythm   Regular
- Ventricular rate   88/min
- Atrial rhythm   None
- Atrial rate   None
- PRI: None
- QRS: 0.12 to 0.14 second

RHYTHM IDENTIFICATION

Monomorphic VT to atrial fibrillation
- Ventricular rhythm   Irregular
- Ventricular rate   214/min (VT) to 71/min (atrial fib)
- Atrial rhythm   Unable to determine
- Atrial rate   Unable to determine
- PRI: Unable to determine
- QRS: 0.12 to 0.16 second (VT) to 0.06 second (atrial fib)

RHYTHM IDENTIFICATION

Sinus rhythm with first-degree AV block and PACs
- Ventricular rhythm   Regular except for the event(s)
- Ventricular rate   79/min (sinus beats)
- Atrial rhythm   Regular except for the event(s)
- Atrial rate   79/min (sinus beats)
- PRI: 0.24 second (sinus beats)
- QRS: 0.08 second (sinus beats)

RHYTHM IDENTIFICATION

Atrial flutter with ST-segment depression
- Ventricular rhythm   Regular
- Ventricular rate   88/min
- Atrial rhythm   Unable to determine
- Atrial rate   Unable to determine
- PRI: Unable to determine
- QRS: 0.06 second

RHYTHM IDENTIFICATION

Second-degree AV block type II with ST-segment depression
- Ventricular rhythm   Irregular
- Ventricular rate   48 to 83/min
- Atrial rhythm   Regular
- Atrial rate   167/min
- PRI: 0.24 second
- QRS: 0.12 second

RHYTHM IDENTIFICATION

Junctional bradycardia with ST-segment depression to sinus bradycardia, inverted T waves
- Ventricular rhythm   Regular
- Ventricular rate   32/min
- Atrial rhythm   None (junctional beats) to regular (sinus beats)
- Atrial rate   32/min (sinus beats)
- PRI: 0.14 second (sinus beats)
- QRS: 0.04 to 0.06 second

RHYTHM IDENTIFICATION

◆ Identify the rhythm.

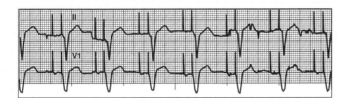

RHYTHM IDENTIFICATION

◆ This rhythm strip is from a 76-year-old man complaining of indigestion. Identify the rhythm (lead II).

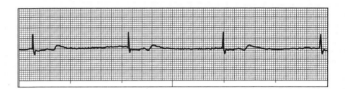

RHYTHM IDENTIFICATION

◆ These rhythm strips are from a 78-year-old man complaining of shortness of breath. He has a history of COPD, coronary artery disease, and hypertension. Identify the rhythm.

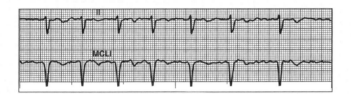

RHYTHM IDENTIFICATION

◆ This rhythm strip is from an 80-year-old woman complaining of weakness. Identify the rhythm (lead II).

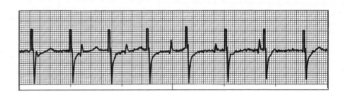

RHYTHM IDENTIFICATION

◆ This rhythm strip is from a 97-year-old woman after a fall. Identify the rhythm (lead II).

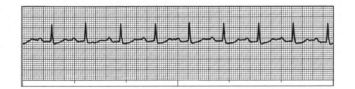

RHYTHM IDENTIFICATION

◆ Identify the rhythm (lead II).

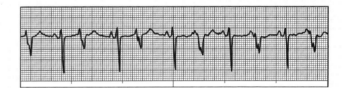

RHYTHM IDENTIFICATION

◆ This rhythm strip is from a 70-year-old man complaining of a sharp pain across his shoulders. Blood pressure 218/86. Identify the rhythm (lead II).

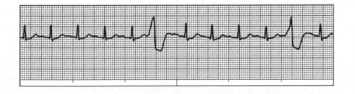

RHYTHM IDENTIFICATION

◆ This rhythm strip is from a 90-year-old woman complaining of hip pain after a fall. Identify the rhythm (lead II).

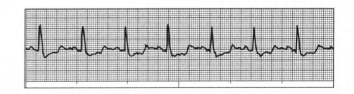

RHYTHM IDENTIFICATION

Junctional bradycardia with ST-segment depression and inverted T waves
- Ventricular rhythm   Regular
- Ventricular rate   32/min
- Atrial rhythm   None
- Atrial rate   None
- PRI: None
- QRS: 0.06 second

RHYTHM IDENTIFICATION

100% paced rhythm—AV sequential pacemaker
- Atrial paced activity?   Yes
- Ventricular paced activity?   Yes
- Paced interval rate?   71

RHYTHM IDENTIFICATION

100% ventricular paced rhythm
- Atrial paced activity?   No
- Ventricular paced activity?   Yes
- Paced interval rate?   83

RHYTHM IDENTIFICATION

Atrial fibrillation (controlled)
- Ventricular rhythm   Irregular
- Ventricular rate   55 to 94/min
- Atrial rhythm   Unable to determine
- Atrial rate   Unable to determine
- PRI: Unable to determine
- QRS: 0.10 second

RHYTHM IDENTIFICATION

Sinus bradycardia with ventricular bigeminy
- Ventricular rhythm   Regular except for the event (every other beat is an ectopic beat)
- Ventricular rate   55/min (sinus beats)
- Atrial rhythm   Regular except for the event (every other beat is an ectopic beat)
- Atrial rate   55/min (sinus beats)
- PRI: 0.12 second (sinus beats)
- QRS: 0.08 to 0.10 second (sinus beats)

RHYTHM IDENTIFICATION

Sinus rhythm with first-degree AV block, ST-segment depression
- Ventricular rhythm   Regular
- Ventricular rate   88/min
- Atrial rhythm   Regular
- Atrial rate   88/min
- PRI: 0.24 second
- QRS: 0.06 second

RHYTHM IDENTIFICATION

Sinus rhythm with ST-segment depression
- Ventricular rhythm   Regular
- Ventricular rate   75/min
- Atrial rhythm   Regular
- Atrial rate   75/min
- PRI: 0.18 second
- QRS: 0.08 to 0.10 second

RHYTHM IDENTIFICATION

Sinus tachycardia with uniform PVCs
- Ventricular rhythm   Regular except for the events
- Ventricular rate   115/min (sinus beats)
- Atrial rhythm   Regular except for the events
- Atrial rate   115/min (sinus beats)
- PRI: 0.18 second (sinus beats)
- QRS: 0.06 second (sinus beats)

RHYTHM IDENTIFICATION

◆ This rhythm strip is from an 86-year-old woman complaining of chest pain that she rates a 4 on a 1 to 10 scale. Blood pressure 142/72. Identify the rhythm.

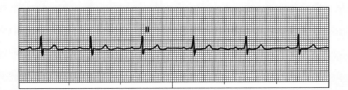

RHYTHM IDENTIFICATION

◆ This rhythm strip is from a 3-month-old infant that had an altered level of responsiveness. She was limp with a respiratory rate of 4 breaths/min. Blood sugar is 174. Identify the rhythm (lead II).

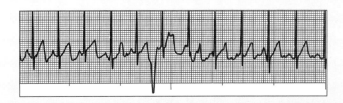

RHYTHM IDENTIFICATION

◆ This rhythm strip is from a 78-year-old man complaining of palpitations. Note the point at which the patient was defibrillated. What is the resulting rhythm?

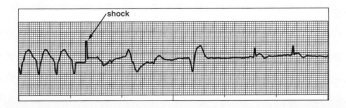

RHYTHM IDENTIFICATION

◆ This rhythm strip is from an 83-year-old man complaining of chest pain. He had a new pacemaker implanted 5 days ago. His blood pressure is 148/60. Identify the rhythm (lead II).

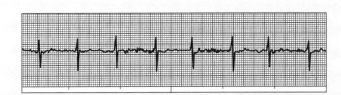

RHYTHM IDENTIFICATION

◆ Identify the rhythm (lead II).

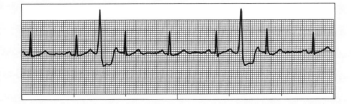

RHYTHM IDENTIFICATION

◆ This rhythm strip is from a 52-year-old man complaining of substernal chest pain. He has a history of COPD and mitral valve regurgitation. Blood pressure 140/78. Identify the rhythm (lead II).

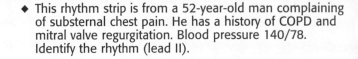

RHYTHM IDENTIFICATION

◆ Identify the rhythm (lead II).

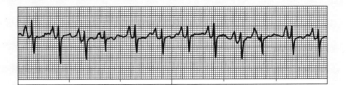

RHYTHM IDENTIFICATION

◆ Identify the rhythm (lead II).

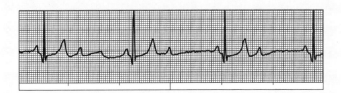

RHYTHM IDENTIFICATION

Sinus tachycardia with an interpolated PVC
- Ventricular rhythm   Regular
- Ventricular rate   125/min
- Atrial rhythm   Regular
- Atrial rate   125/min
- PRI: 0.12 to 0.16 second
- QRS: 0.06 second (sinus beats)

RHYTHM IDENTIFICATION

Sinus rhythm
- Ventricular rhythm   Regular
- Ventricular rate   60/min
- Atrial rhythm   Regular
- Atrial rate   60/min
- PRI: 0.20 second
- QRS: 0.06 second

RHYTHM IDENTIFICATION

Atrial fibrillation (controlled)
- Ventricular rhythm   Regular
- Ventricular rate   79/min
- Atrial rhythm   Unable to determine
- Atrial rate   Unable to determine
- PRI: Unable to determine
- QRS: 0.08 second

RHYTHM IDENTIFICATION

Monomorphic ventricular tachycardia—shock—ventricular beats—sinus arrhythmia
- Ventricular rhythm   Irregular (sinus beats)
- Ventricular rate   63 to 79/min (sinus beats)
- Atrial rhythm   Irregular (sinus beats)
- Atrial rate   63 to 79/min (sinus beats)
- PRI: 0.12 second (sinus beats)
- QRS: 0.04 to 0.06 second (sinus beats)

RHYTHM IDENTIFICATION

Sinus rhythm with ST-segment depression
- Ventricular rhythm   Regular
- Ventricular rate   75/min
- Atrial rhythm   Regular
- Atrial rate   75/min
- PRI: 0.14 second
- QRS: 0.06 to 0.08 second

RHYTHM IDENTIFICATION

Sinus rhythm with uniform PVCs
- Ventricular rhythm   Regular except for the event
- Ventricular rate   68/min (sinus beats)
- Atrial rhythm   Regular except for the event
- Atrial rate   68/min (sinus beats)
- PRI: 0.18 second (sinus beats)
- QRS: 0.06 second (sinus beats)

RHYTHM IDENTIFICATION

Second-degree AV block, 2:1 conduction, probably type I
- Ventricular rhythm   Regular
- Ventricular rate   34/min
- Atrial rhythm   Regular
- Atrial rate   68/min
- PRI: 0.14 to 0.16 second
- QRS: 0.10 second

RHYTHM IDENTIFICATION

Sinus tachycardia with PACs
- Ventricular rhythm   Regular except for the event
- Ventricular rate   115/min (sinus beats)
- Atrial rhythm   Regular except for the event
- Atrial rate   115/min (sinus beats)
- PRI: 0.16 second
- QRS: 0.08 to 0.10 second

RHYTHM IDENTIFICATION

◆ Identify the rhythm (lead II).

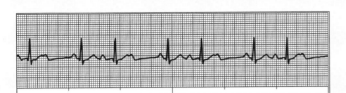

RHYTHM IDENTIFICATION

◆ Identify the rhythm.

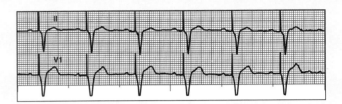

RHYTHM IDENTIFICATION

◆ Identify the rhythm.

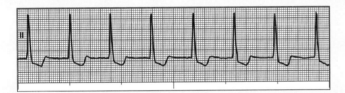

RHYTHM IDENTIFICATION

◆ These rhythm strips are from a 46-year-old woman complaining of abdominal pain. Identify the rhythm.

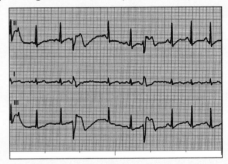

RHYTHM IDENTIFICATION

◆ Identify the rhythm (lead II).

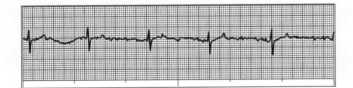

RHYTHM IDENTIFICATION

◆ This rhythm strip is from a 61-year-old man with a history of congestive heart failure. Identify the rhythm.

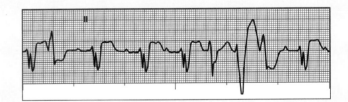

RHYTHM IDENTIFICATION

◆ Identify the rhythm (lead II).

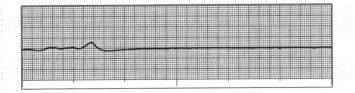

RHYTHM IDENTIFICATION

◆ This rhythm strip is from a 1-month-old infant after a 3-minute seizure. Identify the rhythm (lead II).

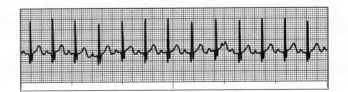

RHYTHM IDENTIFICATION

100% ventricular paced rhythm
- Atrial paced activity?   No
- Ventricular paced activity?   Yes
- Paced interval rate?   65

RHYTHM IDENTIFICATION

Second-degree AV block, type I
- Ventricular rhythm   Irregular
- Ventricular rate   60 to 98/min
- Atrial rhythm   Regular
- Atrial rate   111/min
- PRI: Lengthens
- QRS: 0.08 second

RHYTHM IDENTIFICATION

Sinus tachycardia with uniform PVCs
- Ventricular rhythm   Regular except for the events
- Ventricular rate   107/min (sinus beats)
- Atrial rhythm   Regular except for the events
- Atrial rate   107/min (sinus beats)
- PRI: 0.14 second (sinus beats)
- QRS: 0.06 second (sinus beats)

RHYTHM IDENTIFICATION

Accelerated junctional rhythm
- Ventricular rhythm   Regular
- Ventricular rate   75/min
- Atrial rhythm   None
- Atrial rate   None
- PRI: None
- QRS: 0.08 second

RHYTHM IDENTIFICATION

Sinus rhythm with first-degree AV block, wide QRS (bundle branch block), multiform PVCs, and ST-segment elevation
- Ventricular rhythm   Irregular
- Ventricular rate   65 to 75/min (sinus beats)
- Atrial rhythm   Irregular
- Atrial rate   65 to 75/min (sinus beats)
- PRI: 0.32 second (sinus beats)
- QRS: 0.18 second (sinus beats)

RHYTHM IDENTIFICATION

Atrial fibrillation (controlled)
- Ventricular rhythm   Regular
- Ventricular rate   54/min
- Atrial rhythm   Unable to determine
- Atrial rate   Unable to determine
- PRI: Unable to determine
- QRS: 0.08 second

RHYTHM IDENTIFICATION

Sinus tachycardia
- Ventricular rhythm   Regular
- Ventricular rate   130/min
- Atrial rhythm   Regular
- Atrial rate   130/min
- PRI: 0.14 to 0.16 second
- QRS: 0.06 to 0.08 second

RHYTHM IDENTIFICATION

Asystole
- Ventricular rhythm   None
- Ventricular rate   None
- Atrial rhythm   None
- Atrial rate   None
- PRI: None
- QRS: None

RHYTHM IDENTIFICATION

◆ Identify the rhythm.

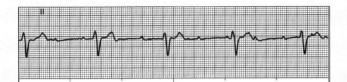

RHYTHM IDENTIFICATION

◆ Identify the rhythm (lead II).

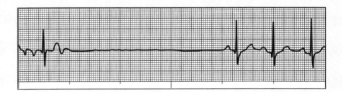

RHYTHM IDENTIFICATION

◆ This rhythm strip is from a 72-year-old man complaining of chest pain. Identify the rhythm (lead I).

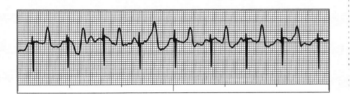

RHYTHM IDENTIFICATION

◆ Identify the rhythm (lead II).

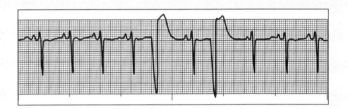

RHYTHM IDENTIFICATION

◆ This rhythm strip is from a 77-year-old woman with a congested cough. Identify the rhythm (lead II).

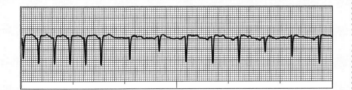

RHYTHM IDENTIFICATION

◆ This rhythm strip is from a 54-year-old man who had a syncopal episode. Identify the rhythm.

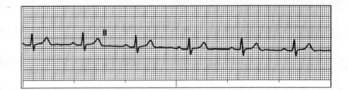

RHYTHM IDENTIFICATION

◆ Identify the rhythm (lead II).

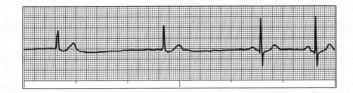

RHYTHM IDENTIFICATION

◆ This rhythm strip is from a 66-year-old man complaining of chest pain. Blood pressure 170/96. Identify the rhythm (lead II).

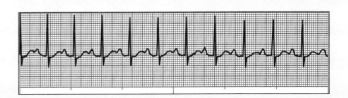

RHYTHM IDENTIFICATION

Atrial flutter to sinus rhythm
- ◆ Ventricular rhythm   Regular (sinus beats)
- ◆ Ventricular rate   83/min (sinus beats)
- ◆ Atrial rhythm   Regular (sinus beats)
- ◆ Atrial rate   83/min (sinus beats)
- ◆ PRI: 0.20 second (sinus beats)
- ◆ QRS: 0.06 to 0.08 second (sinus beats)

RHYTHM IDENTIFICATION

Complete (third-degree) AV block
- ◆ Ventricular rhythm   Regular
- ◆ Ventricular rate   45/min
- ◆ Atrial rhythm   Regular
- ◆ Atrial rate   115/min
- ◆ PRI: Varies
- ◆ QRS: 0.16 second

RHYTHM IDENTIFICATION

Sinus rhythm with uniform PVCs
- ◆ Ventricular rhythm   Regular except for the event
- ◆ Ventricular rate   96/min (sinus beats)
- ◆ Atrial rhythm   Regular except for the event
- ◆ Atrial rate   96/min (sinus beats)
- ◆ PRI: 0.12 second (sinus beats)
- ◆ QRS: 0.08 to 0.10 second (sinus beats)

RHYTHM IDENTIFICATION

100% ventricular paced rhythm
- ◆ Atrial paced activity?   No
- ◆ Ventricular paced activity?   Yes
- ◆ Paced interval rate?   60

RHYTHM IDENTIFICATION

Sinus bradycardia
- ◆ Ventricular rhythm   Regular
- ◆ Ventricular rate   58/min
- ◆ Atrial rhythm   Regular
- ◆ Atrial rate   58/min
- ◆ PRI: 0.20 second
- ◆ QRS: 0.08 second

RHYTHM IDENTIFICATION

Atrial fibrillation (uncontrolled)
- ◆ Ventricular rhythm   Irregular
- ◆ Ventricular rate   107 to 200/min
- ◆ Atrial rhythm   Unable to determine
- ◆ Atrial rate   Unable to determine
- ◆ PRI: Unable to determine
- ◆ QRS: 0.06 to 0.08 second

RHYTHM IDENTIFICATION

Sinus tachycardia with first-degree AV block
- ◆ Ventricular rhythm   Regular
- ◆ Ventricular rate   107/min
- ◆ Atrial rhythm   Regular
- ◆ Atrial rate   107/min
- ◆ PRI: 0.24 second
- ◆ QRS: 0.08 second

RHYTHM IDENTIFICATION

Junctional bradycardia to sinus bradycardia
- ◆ Ventricular rhythm   Irregular (junctional beats) to regular (sinus beats)
- ◆ Ventricular rate   30/min (junctional beats) to 56/min (sinus beats)
- ◆ Atrial rhythm   None (junctional beats) to regular (sinus beats)
- ◆ Atrial rate   None (junctional beats) to 56/min (sinus beats)
- ◆ PRI: None (junctional beats) to 0.18 second (sinus beats)
- ◆ QRS: 0.04 (junctional beats) to 0.08 second (sinus beats)

RHYTHM IDENTIFICATION

◆ This rhythm strip is from a 43-year-old woman complaining of palpitations. Identify the rhythm (lead II).

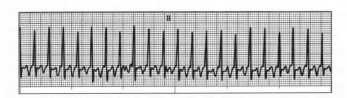

RHYTHM IDENTIFICATION

◆ Identify the rhythm (lead II).

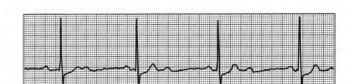

RHYTHM IDENTIFICATION

◆ A 43-year-old woman is complaining of palpitations. The patient has a history of SVT and states she cannot tolerate adenosine. The following rhythm is observed on the cardiac monitor after diltiazem administration. Identify the rhythm.

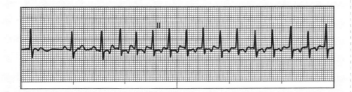

RHYTHM IDENTIFICATION

◆ This rhythm strip is from a 74-year-old woman complaining of difficulty breathing. Blood pressure 158/122. Identify the rhythm (lead II).

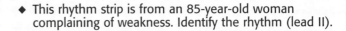
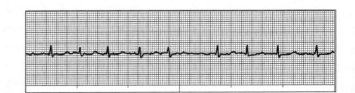

RHYTHM IDENTIFICATION

◆ Identify the rhythm (lead II).

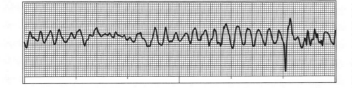

RHYTHM IDENTIFICATION

◆ This rhythm strip is from an 85-year-old woman complaining of weakness. Identify the rhythm (lead II).

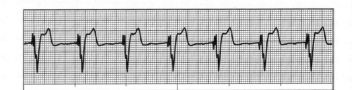

RHYTHM IDENTIFICATION

◆ Identify the rhythm (lead II).

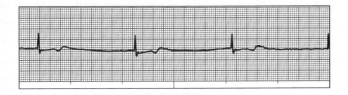

RHYTHM IDENTIFICATION

◆ This rhythm strip is from a 78-year-old man complaining of palpitations. Identify the rhythm.

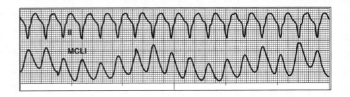

RHYTHM IDENTIFICATION

Second-degree AV block, 2:1 conduction, probably type I;
ST-segment depression
- ◆ Ventricular rhythm   Regular
- ◆ Ventricular rate   38/min
- ◆ Atrial rhythm   Regular
- ◆ Atrial rate   76/min
- ◆ PRI: 0.20 to 0.24 second
- ◆ QRS: 0.08 to 0.10 second

RHYTHM IDENTIFICATION

Narrow-QRS tachycardia
- ◆ Ventricular rhythm   Regular
- ◆ Ventricular rate   214/min
- ◆ Atrial rhythm   Unable to determine
- ◆ Atrial rate   Unable to determine
- ◆ PRI: Unable to determine
- ◆ QRS: 0.08 second

RHYTHM IDENTIFICATION

Atrial fibrillation
- ◆ Ventricular rhythm   Irregular
- ◆ Ventricular rate   65 to 103/min
- ◆ Atrial rhythm   Unable to determine
- ◆ Atrial rate   Unable to determine
- ◆ PRI: Unable to determine
- ◆ QRS: 0.06 to 0.08 second

RHYTHM IDENTIFICATION

Junctional to sinus to narrow-QRS tachycardia
- ◆ Ventricular rhythm   Regular (atrial beats)
- ◆ Ventricular rate   187/min (atrial beats)
- ◆ Atrial rhythm   Unable to determine
- ◆ Atrial rate   Unable to determine
- ◆ PRI: Unable to determine
- ◆ QRS: 0.08 second (atrial beats)

RHYTHM IDENTIFICATION

100% ventricular paced rhythm
- ◆ Atrial paced activity?   No
- ◆ Ventricular paced activity? Yes
- ◆ Paced interval rate?   70

RHYTHM IDENTIFICATION

Ventricular fibrillation (coarse)
- ◆ Ventricular rhythm   Unable to determine
- ◆ Ventricular rate   Unable to determine
- ◆ Atrial rhythm   Unable to determine
- ◆ Atrial rate   Unable to determine
- ◆ PRI: Unable to determine
- ◆ QRS: Unable to determine

RHYTHM IDENTIFICATION

Monomorphic ventricular tachycardia
- ◆ Ventricular rhythm   Regular
- ◆ Ventricular rate   167/min
- ◆ Atrial rhythm   Unable to determine
- ◆ Atrial rate   Unable to determine
- ◆ PRI: Unable to determine
- ◆ QRS: 0.16 second

RHYTHM IDENTIFICATION

Junctional bradycardia with ST-segment depression
- ◆ Ventricular rhythm   Regular
- ◆ Ventricular rate   32/min
- ◆ Atrial rhythm   None
- ◆ Atrial rate   None
- ◆ PRI: None
- ◆ QRS: 0.06 to 0.08 second

RHYTHM IDENTIFICATION

- Identify the rhythm (lead II).

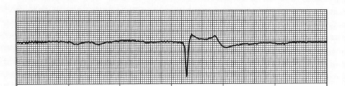

RHYTHM IDENTIFICATION

- This rhythm strip is from an 83-year-old woman complaining of shortness of breath. Identify the rhythm (top = lead II, bottom = lead V₁).

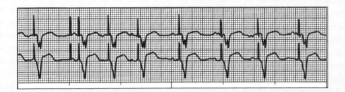

RHYTHM IDENTIFICATION

- This rhythm strip is from a 17-year-old male that experienced a syncopal episode while playing baseball in 110°F heat for 4 hours. Blood pressure 148/84. Core temperature 101.8°F. Identify the rhythm (lead II).

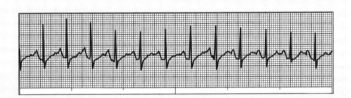

RHYTHM IDENTIFICATION

- This rhythm strip is from a 78-year-old man with chest pain. Identify the rhythm (lead II).

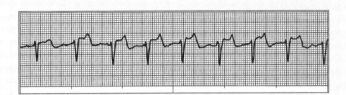

RHYTHM IDENTIFICATION

- Identify the rhythm (lead II).

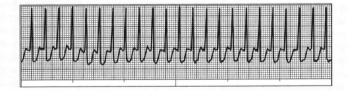

RHYTHM IDENTIFICATION

- These rhythm strips are from a 78-year-old woman complaining of shortness of breath. Identify the rhythm.

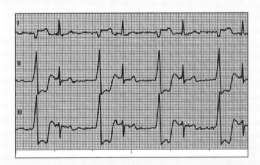

RHYTHM IDENTIFICATION

- These rhythm strips are from a 35-year-old man reporting a sudden onset of severe substernal chest pain. He has no significant medical history and takes no medications. His initial blood pressure is 56/0. Identify the rhythm.

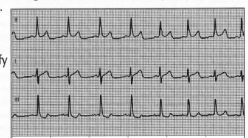

RHYTHM IDENTIFICATION

- Identify the rhythm.

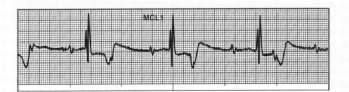

AV sequential demand pacemaker
- Atrial paced activity?   Yes
- Ventricular paced activity?   Yes
- Paced interval rate?   Atrial = 79, ventricular = 100

Ventricular escape beat/asystole
- Ventricular rhythm   None
- Ventricular rate   None
- Atrial rhythm   None
- Atrial rate   None
- PRI: None
- QRS: 0.12 second

Atrial fibrillation
- Ventricular rhythm   Irregular
- Ventricular rate   94 to 100/min
- Atrial rhythm   Unable to determine
- Atrial rate   Unable to determine
- PRI: Unable to determine
- QRS: 0.10 second

Sinus tachycardia
- Ventricular rhythm   Regular
- Ventricular rate   125/min
- Atrial rhythm   Regular
- Atrial rate   125/min
- PRI: 0.16 second
- QRS: 0.06 second

Sinus bradycardia with ventricular bigeminy
- Ventricular rhythm   Regular except for the event (every other beat is an ectopic beat)
- Ventricular rate   40/min (sinus beats)
- Atrial rhythm   Regular except for the event
- Atrial rate   40/min (sinus beats)
- PRI: 0.08 to 0.12 second (sinus beats)
- QRS: 0.08 second (sinus beats)

Narrow-QRS tachycardia (supraventricular tachycardia [SVT]) with ST-segment depression
- Ventricular rhythm   Regular
- Ventricular rate   231/min
- Atrial rhythm   Unable to determine
- Atrial rate   Unable to determine
- PRI: Unable to determine
- QRS: 0.06 second

Complete (third-degree) AV block
- Ventricular rhythm   Regular
- Ventricular rate   37/min
- Atrial rhythm   Regular
- Atrial rate   79/min
- PRI: Varies
- QRS: 0.12 to 0.14 second

Sinus rhythm
- Ventricular rhythm   Regular
- Ventricular rate   71/min
- Atrial rhythm   Regular
- Atrial rate   71/min
- PRI: 0.14 second
- QRS: 0.08 second

◆ This rhythm strip is from an 18-year-old male with a gunshot wound to his chest. Identify the rhythm (lead II).

◆ This rhythm strip is from an 84-year-old man complaining of dizziness. He had a triple bypass 4 days ago. Identify the rhythm (lead II).

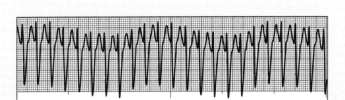

◆ Identify the rhythm.

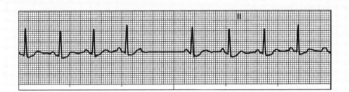

◆ Identify the rhythm (lead II).

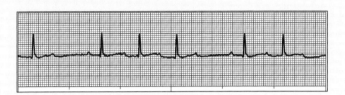

◆ Identify the rhythm (lead II).

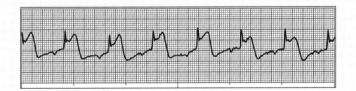

◆ Identify the rhythm (lead II).

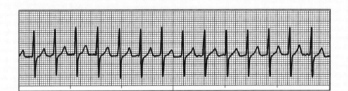

◆ Identify the rhythm (lead II).

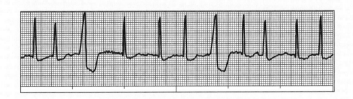

◆ The following rhythm is observed on the cardiac monitor after administration of 6 mg adenosine IV. Identify the rhythm (lead II).

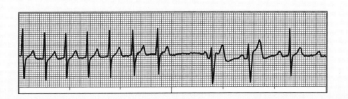

RHYTHM IDENTIFICATION

Monomorphic ventricular tachycardia
- Ventricular rhythm   Regular
- Ventricular rate   214/min
- Atrial rhythm   Unable to determine
- Atrial rate   Unable to determine
- PRI: Unable to determine
- QRS: 0.14 second

Note: This rhythm converted to a sinus rhythm after administration of IV lidocaine.

RHYTHM IDENTIFICATION

Agonal/asystole
- Ventricular rhythm   None
- Ventricular rate   None
- Atrial rhythm   None
- Atrial rate   None
- PRI: None
- QRS: 0.28 second

RHYTHM IDENTIFICATION

Second-degree AV block type 1
- Ventricular rhythm   Irregular
- Ventricular rate   51 to 83/min
- Atrial rhythm   Regular
- Atrial rate   88/min
- PRI: Lengthens
- QRS: 0.06 second

RHYTHM IDENTIFICATION

Sinus rhythm with a nonconducted PAC
- Ventricular rhythm   Regular except for the event
- Ventricular rate   91/min
- Atrial rhythm   Regular except for the event
- Atrial rate   91/min
- PRI: 0.16 second
- QRS: 0.06 second

RHYTHM IDENTIFICATION

Narrow-QRS tachycardia (supraventricular tachycardia [SVT])
- Ventricular rhythm   Regular
- Ventricular rate   150/min
- Atrial rhythm   Unable to determine
- Atrial rate   Unable to determine
- PRI: Unable to determine
- QRS: 0.08 second

RHYTHM IDENTIFICATION

Accelerated junctional rhythm with ST-segment elevation
- Ventricular rhythm   Regular
- Ventricular rate   71/min
- Atrial rhythm   Regular
- Atrial rate   71/min
- PRI: 0.14 second
- QRS: 0.08 second

RHYTHM IDENTIFICATION

Conversion from narrow-QRS tachycardia to sinus rhythm
- Ventricular rhythm   Irregular
- Ventricular rate   130/min (narrow-QRS tach) to 75/min (sinus beats)
- Atrial rhythm   Irregular
- Atrial rate   Unable to determine (narrow-QRS tach) to 75/min (sinus beats)
- PRI: 0.24 second (last sinus beat)
- QRS: 0.08 second (last sinus beat)

RHYTHM IDENTIFICATION

Atrial fibrillation with uniform ventricular complexes
- Ventricular rhythm   Irregular
- Ventricular rate   88 to 167/min
- Atrial rhythm   Unable to determine
- Atrial rate   Unable to determine
- PRI: Unable to determine
- QRS: 0.06 to 0.08 second

RHYTHM IDENTIFICATION

◆ Identify the rhythm (lead II).

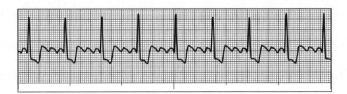

RHYTHM IDENTIFICATION

◆ Identify the rhythm (lead II).

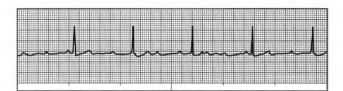

RHYTHM IDENTIFICATION

◆ Identify the rhythm (lead II).

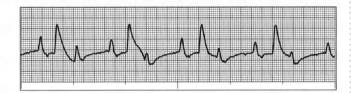

RHYTHM IDENTIFICATION

◆ This rhythm strip is from a 79-year-old woman with epistaxis. Blood pressure 222/118. Identify the rhythm (lead II).

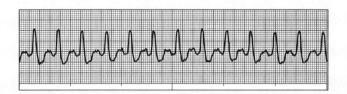

RHYTHM IDENTIFICATION

◆ Identify the rhythm.

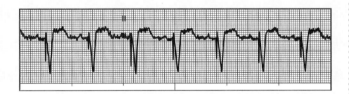

RHYTHM IDENTIFICATION

◆ This rhythm strip is from an 84-year-old woman complaining of chest pain. Blood pressure 140/54. Identify the rhythm (lead III).

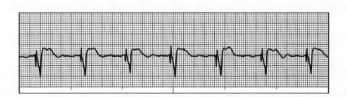

RHYTHM IDENTIFICATION

◆ Identify the rhythm (lead II).

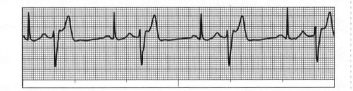

RHYTHM IDENTIFICATION

◆ Identify the rhythm (lead II).

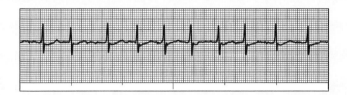

RHYTHM IDENTIFICATION

Complete (third-degree) AV block
- Ventricular rhythm — Regular
- Ventricular rate — 53/min
- Atrial rhythm — Regular
- Atrial rate — 136/min
- PRI: — Varies
- QRS: — 0.04 to 0.06 second

RHYTHM IDENTIFICATION

Atrial flutter with ST-segment depression
- Ventricular rhythm — Regular
- Ventricular rate — 88/min
- Atrial rhythm — Unable to determine
- Atrial rate — Unable to determine
- PRI: — Unable to determine
- QRS: — 0.06 to 0.08 second

RHYTHM IDENTIFICATION

Sinus tachycardia with a wide-QRS and ST-segment depression
- Ventricular rhythm — Regular
- Ventricular rate — 130/min
- Atrial rhythm — Regular
- Atrial rate — 130/min
- PRI: — 0.16 second
- QRS: — 0.12 second

RHYTHM IDENTIFICATION

Complete (third-degree) AV block with ST-segment depression
- Ventricular rhythm — Regular
- Ventricular rate — 34/min
- Atrial rhythm — Regular
- Atrial rate — 88/min
- PRI: — Varies
- QRS: — 0.16 second

RHYTHM IDENTIFICATION

100% ventricular paced rhythm
- Atrial paced activity? — No
- Ventricular paced activity? — Yes
- Paced interval rate? — 68

RHYTHM IDENTIFICATION

100% ventricular paced rhythm
- Atrial paced activity? — No
- Ventricular paced activity? — Yes
- Paced interval rate? — 78

RHYTHM IDENTIFICATION

Atrial fibrillation
- Ventricular rhythm — Irregular
- Ventricular rate — 70 to 103/min
- Atrial rhythm — Unable to determine
- Atrial rate — Unable to determine
- PRI: — Unable to determine
- QRS: — 0.06 second

RHYTHM IDENTIFICATION

Sinus bradycardia with ventricular bigeminy
- Ventricular rhythm — Regular except for the event (every other beat is an ectopic beat)
- Ventricular rate — 36/min (sinus beats)
- Atrial rhythm — Regular except for the event
- Atrial rate — 36/min (sinus beats)
- PRI: — 0.16 to 0.18 second (sinus beats)
- QRS: — 0.04 to 0.06 second (sinus beats)

RHYTHM IDENTIFICATION

- ♦ !dentify the rhythm (lead II).

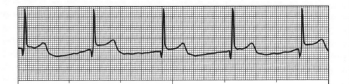

RHYTHM IDENTIFICATION

- ♦ These rhythm strips are from a 58-year-old man complaining of palpitations. Identify the rhythm.

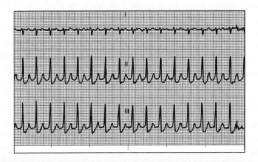

RHYTHM IDENTIFICATION

- ♦ This rhythm strip is from a 52-year-old man found unresponsive, apneic, and pulseless. Identify the rhythm (lead II).

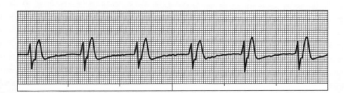

RHYTHM IDENTIFICATION

- ♦ These rhythm strips are from a 58-year-old man complaining of palpitations, 40 seconds after administration of 6 mg adenosine IV. Identify the rhythm.

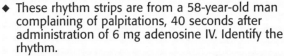
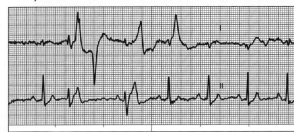

RHYTHM IDENTIFICATION

- ♦ This rhythm strip is from a 6-year-old girl complaining of abdominal pain. Blood pressure 100/60. Identify the rhythm.

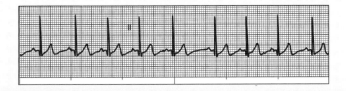

RHYTHM IDENTIFICATION

- ♦ Identify the rhythm (lead II).

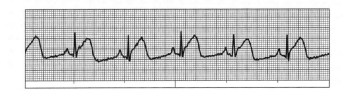
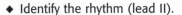

RHYTHM IDENTIFICATION

- ♦ Identify the rhythm.

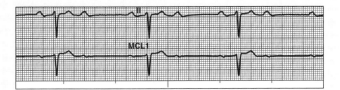

RHYTHM IDENTIFICATION

- ♦ Identify the rhythm.

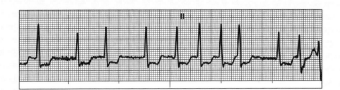

RHYTHM IDENTIFICATION

Narrow-QRS tachycardia (supraventricular tachycardia [SVT]) with ST-segment depression
- Ventricular rhythm — Regular
- Ventricular rate — 167/min
- Atrial rhythm — Unable to determine
- Atrial rate — Unable to determine
- PRI: — Unable to determine
- QRS: — 0.06 second

RHYTHM IDENTIFICATION

Junctional escape rhythm
- Ventricular rhythm — Regular
- Ventricular rate — 45/min
- Atrial rhythm — None
- Atrial rate — None
- PRI: — None
- QRS: — 0.08 second

RHYTHM IDENTIFICATION

Conversion from narrow-QRS tachycardia to sinus rhythm with first-degree AV block
- Ventricular rhythm — Regular (sinus beats)
- Ventricular rate — 75/min (sinus beats)
- Atrial rhythm — Regular (sinus beats)
- Atrial rate — 75/min (sinus beats)
- PRI: — 0.24 second (sinus beats)
- QRS: — 0.06 second (sinus beats)

RHYTHM IDENTIFICATION

Accelerated idioventricular rhythm (AIVR)
- Ventricular rhythm — Regular
- Ventricular rate — 60/min
- Atrial rhythm — Unable to determine
- Atrial rate — Unable to determine
- PRI: — Unable to determine
- QRS: — 0.12 to 0.14 second

RHYTHM IDENTIFICATION

Sinus bradycardia with ST-segment elevation and tall T waves
- Ventricular rhythm — Regular
- Ventricular rate — 58/min
- Atrial rhythm — Regular
- Atrial rate — 58/min
- PRI: — 0.16 second
- QRS: — 0.08 second

RHYTHM IDENTIFICATION

Sinus arrhythmia
- Ventricular rhythm — Irregular
- Ventricular rate — 75 to 100/min
- Atrial rhythm — Irregular
- Atrial rate — 75 to 100/min
- PRI: — 0.14 to 0.16 second
- QRS: — 0.08 second

RHYTHM IDENTIFICATION

Atrial fibrillation with ST-segment depression
- Ventricular rhythm — Irregular
- Ventricular rate — 75 to 176/min
- Atrial rhythm — Unable to determine
- Atrial rate — Unable to determine
- PRI: — Unable to determine
- QRS: — 0.08 to 0.10 second

RHYTHM IDENTIFICATION

Second-degree AV block, 2:1 conduction, probably type I
- Ventricular rhythm — Regular
- Ventricular rate — 36/min
- Atrial rhythm — Regular
- Atrial rate — 72/min
- PRI: — 0.32 second
- QRS: — 0.10 second

RHYTHM IDENTIFICATION

◆ Identify the rhythm.

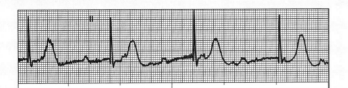

RHYTHM IDENTIFICATION

◆ Identify the rhythm (lead II).

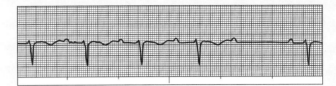

RHYTHM IDENTIFICATION

◆ Identify the rhythm.

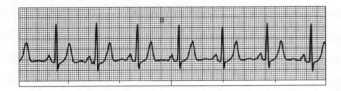

RHYTHM IDENTIFICATION

◆ This rhythm strip is from a 43-year-old man after a seizure. Identify the rhythm (lead II).

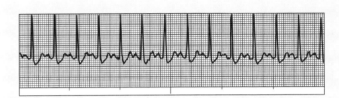

RHYTHM IDENTIFICATION

◆ Identify the rhythm (lead II).

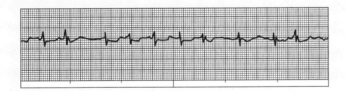

RHYTHM IDENTIFICATION

◆ This rhythm strip is from an 84-year-old man complaining of dizziness. He had a triple bypass 4 days ago. Identify the rhythm (lead II).

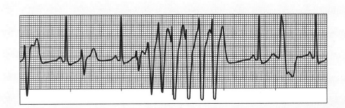

RHYTHM IDENTIFICATION

◆ This rhythm strip is from an 87-year-old woman complaining of weakness. Identify the rhythm (lead II).

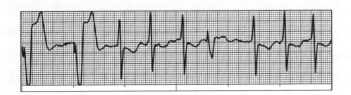

RHYTHM IDENTIFICATION

◆ This rhythm strip is from a 44-year-old construction worker complaining of a sudden onset of chest pressure. Identify the rhythm (lead II).

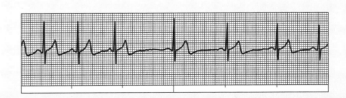

Second-degree AV block type II
- Ventricular rhythm   Irregular
- Ventricular rate   28 to 55/min
- Atrial rhythm   Regular
- Atrial rate   55/min
- PRI: 0.40 second
- QRS: 0.12 second

Complete (third-degree) AV block
- Ventricular rhythm   Regular
- Ventricular rate   37/min
- Atrial rhythm   Regular
- Atrial rate   81/min
- PRI: Varies
- QRS: 0.10 second

Sinus tachycardia with ST-segment depression
- Ventricular rhythm   Regular
- Ventricular rate   107/min
- Atrial rhythm   Regular
- Atrial rate   107/min
- PRI: 0.18 second
- QRS: 0.08 second

Sinus rhythm with tall T waves
- Ventricular rhythm   Regular
- Ventricular rate   72/min
- Atrial rhythm   Regular
- Atrial rate   72/min
- PRI: 0.16 second
- QRS: 0.08 second

Sinus bradycardia with ventricular bigeminy and a run of VT, ST-segment depression
- Ventricular rhythm   Irregular
- Ventricular rate   56/min (sinus beats)
- Atrial rhythm   Irregular (sinus beats)
- Atrial rate   56/min (sinus beats)
- PRI: 0.16 second (sinus beats)
- QRS: 0.06 second (sinus beats)

Atrial fibrillation
- Ventricular rhythm   Irregular
- Ventricular rate   77 to 150/min
- Atrial rhythm   Unable to determine
- Atrial rate   Unable to determine
- PRI: Unable to determine
- QRS: 0.08 second

Sinus arrhythmia
- Ventricular rhythm   Irregular
- Ventricular rate   52 to 94/min
- Atrial rhythm   Irregular
- Atrial rate   52 to 94/min
- PRI: 0.12 second
- QRS: 0.08 second

Ventricular demand pacemaker
- Atrial paced activity?   No
- Ventricular paced activity?   Yes
- Paced interval rate?   62

RHYTHM IDENTIFICATION

◆ These rhythm strips are from a 41-year-old woman complaining of generalized abdominal pain. Identify the rhythm.

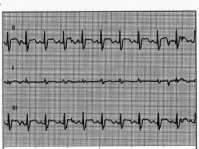

RHYTHM IDENTIFICATION

◆ Identify the rhythm (lead II).

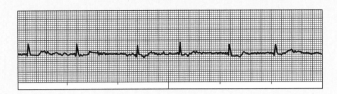

RHYTHM IDENTIFICATION

◆ This rhythm strip is from a 67-year-old woman with a decreased level of responsiveness. Identify the rhythm (lead II).

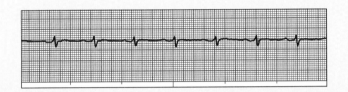

RHYTHM IDENTIFICATION

◆ Identify the rhythm (lead II).

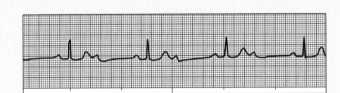

RHYTHM IDENTIFICATION

◆ This rhythm strip is from a 47-year-old woman complaining of a sudden onset of left arm weakness/numbness while sitting at her desk. Identify the rhythm.

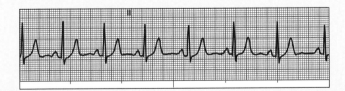

RHYTHM IDENTIFICATION

◆ Identify the rhythm (lead II).

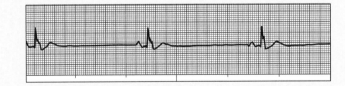

RHYTHM IDENTIFICATION

◆ This rhythm strip is from a 77-year-old woman complaining of weakness and dizziness. Identify the rhythm (lead II).

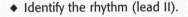
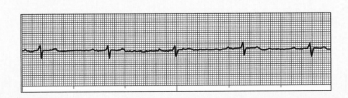

RHYTHM IDENTIFICATION

◆ This rhythm strip is from a 76-year-old woman complaining of back pain. She states she had a myocardial infarction 2 years ago. Identify the rhythm (lead II).

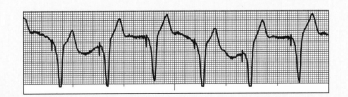

RHYTHM IDENTIFICATION

Atrial fibrillation (controlled)
- Ventricular rhythm   Irregular
- Ventricular rate   50 to 71/min
- Atrial rhythm   Unable to determine
- Atrial rate   Unable to determine
- PRI: Unable to determine
- QRS: 0.08 to 0.10 second

RHYTHM IDENTIFICATION

Sinus tachycardia
- Ventricular rhythm   Regular
- Ventricular rate   Approximately 110/min
- Atrial rhythm   Regular
- Atrial rate   Approximately 110/min
- PRI: 0.18 second
- QRS: 0.06 second

RHYTHM IDENTIFICATION

Second-degree AV block, 2:1 conduction, probably type I
- Ventricular rhythm   Regular
- Ventricular rate   37/min
- Atrial rhythm   Regular
- Atrial rate   75/min
- PRI: 0.28 second
- QRS: 0.06 second

RHYTHM IDENTIFICATION

Sinus rhythm with first-degree AV block
- Ventricular rhythm   Regular
- Ventricular rate   Approximately 75/min
- Atrial rhythm   Regular
- Atrial rate   Approximately 75/min
- PRI: 0.24 second
- QRS: 0.10 second

RHYTHM IDENTIFICATION

Sinus bradycardia with first-degree AV block, wide-QRS (probable bundle branch block), ST-segment depression
- Ventricular rhythm   Regular
- Ventricular rate   27/min
- Atrial rhythm   Regular
- Atrial rate   27/min
- PRI: 0.22 second
- QRS: 0.12 second

RHYTHM IDENTIFICATION

Sinus rhythm (with tall T waves)
- Ventricular rhythm   Regular
- Ventricular rate   70/min
- Atrial rhythm   Regular
- Atrial rate   70/min
- PRI: 0.18 second
- QRS: 0.08 to 0.10 second

RHYTHM IDENTIFICATION

100% ventricular paced rhythm
- Atrial paced activity?   No
- Ventricular paced activity?   Yes
- Paced interval rate?   65

RHYTHM IDENTIFICATION

Sinus bradycardia with first-degree AV block
- Ventricular rhythm   Regular
- Ventricular rate   46/min
- Atrial rhythm   Regular
- Atrial rate   46/min
- PRI: 0.24 to 0.28 second
- QRS: 0.08 second

Note: Patient's potassium level was 7.0. A permanent pacemaker was inserted.

RHYTHM IDENTIFICATION

◆ This rhythm strip is from an 80-year-old man found sitting in a chair. He is unresponsive, apneic, and pulseless. Identify the rhythm (lead II).

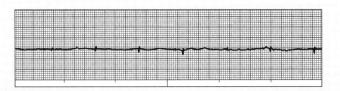

RHYTHM IDENTIFICATION

◆ This rhythm strip is from an 88-year-old woman complaining of hip pain after a fall injury. Identify the rhythm (lead II).

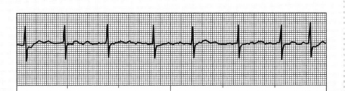

RHYTHM IDENTIFICATION

◆ Identify the rhythm.

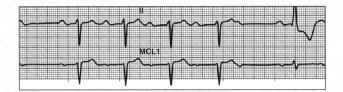

RHYTHM IDENTIFICATION

◆ Identify the rhythm (lead II).

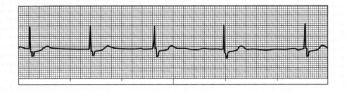

RHYTHM IDENTIFICATION

◆ This rhythm strip is from a 67-year-old woman found unresponsive on the side of the road. Outdoor temperature 112° F. Blood pressure 238/110, respiratory rate 60/min. Identify the rhythm (lead II).

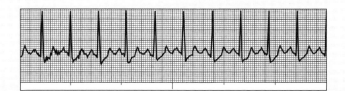

RHYTHM IDENTIFICATION

◆ This rhythm strip is from an 84-year-old man complaining of dizziness. He had a triple bypass 4 days ago. Identify the rhythm (lead II).

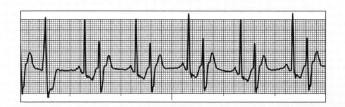

RHYTHM IDENTIFICATION

◆ This rhythm strip is from an 81-year-old woman with an altered level of responsiveness. Blood pressure 160/70. Blood sugar 114. Identify the rhythm.

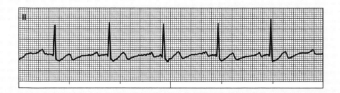

RHYTHM IDENTIFICATION

◆ This rhythm strip is from a 80-year-old woman who was playing Bingo when she felt dizzy and slumped over in her chair. Bystanders state she was unresponsive for approximately 5 minutes. A pulse is present. Identify the rhythm.

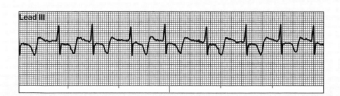

RHYTHM IDENTIFICATION

Sinus tachycardia with ST-segment depression
- Ventricular rhythm   Regular
- Ventricular rate   136/min
- Atrial rhythm   Regular
- Atrial rate   136/min
- PRI: 0.16 second
- QRS: 0.08 second

RHYTHM IDENTIFICATION

Asystole—the electrical activity shown is due to pacemaker spikes from the patient's permanent pacemaker (no capture).
- Ventricular rhythm   None
- Ventricular rate   None
- Atrial rhythm   None
- Atrial rate   None
- PRI: None
- QRS: None

RHYTHM IDENTIFICATION

Sinus rhythm with ventricular bigeminy, ST-segment depression
- Ventricular rhythm   Regular except for the event (every other beat is an ectopic beat)
- Ventricular rate   60/min (sinus beats)
- Atrial rhythm   Regular except for the event
- Atrial rate   60/min (sinus beats)
- PRI: 0.16 second (sinus beats)
- QRS: 0.08 second (sinus beats)

RHYTHM IDENTIFICATION

Atrial fibrillation
- Ventricular rhythm   Irregular
- Ventricular rate   68 to 125/min
- Atrial rhythm   Unable to determine
- Atrial rate   Unable to determine
- PRI: Unable to determine
- QRS: 0.08 second

RHYTHM IDENTIFICATION

Sinus bradycardia with a first-degree AV block
- Ventricular rhythm   Regular
- Ventricular rate   56/min
- Atrial rhythm   Regular
- Atrial rate   56/min
- PRI: 0.24 second
- QRS: 0.06 second

RHYTHM IDENTIFICATION

Second-degree AV block type I with a ventricular complex
- Ventricular rhythm   Irregular
- Ventricular rate   42 to 68/min
- Atrial rhythm   Regular
- Atrial rate   68/min
- PRI: Lengthens
- QRS: 0.10 second

RHYTHM IDENTIFICATION

Atrial fibrillation (controlled)
- Ventricular rhythm   Irregular
- Ventricular rate   75 to 94/min
- Atrial rhythm   Unable to determine
- Atrial rate   Unable to determine
- PRI: Unable to determine
- QRS: 0.08 second

RHYTHM IDENTIFICATION

Sinus bradycardia with a first-degree AV block to junctional escape rhythm
- Ventricular rhythm   Regular (junctional beats)
- Ventricular rate   48/min (junctional beats)
- Atrial rhythm   Unable to determine (junctional beats)
- Atrial rate   Unable to determine (junctional beats)
- PRI: Unable to determine (junctional beats)
- QRS: 0.06 to 0.08 second

RHYTHM IDENTIFICATION

◆ This rhythm strip is from a 91-year-old woman complaining of chest pain and difficulty breathing. Identify the rhythm (lead II).

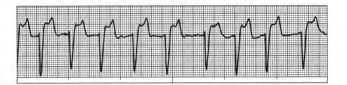

RHYTHM IDENTIFICATION

◆ This rhythm strip is from a 62-year-old woman complaining of chest pain. Her blood pressure is 146/104, respirations 20. Breath sounds are clear. Identify the rhythm (lead II).

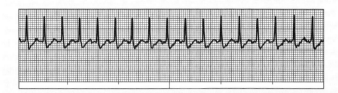

RHYTHM IDENTIFICATION

◆ This rhythm strip is from an 85-year-old woman complaining of numbness in her legs. Identify the rhythm (lead II).

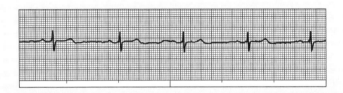

RHYTHM IDENTIFICATION

◆ This rhythm strip is from a 6-year-old boy immediately after a seizure. Identify the rhythm (lead II).

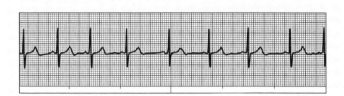

RHYTHM IDENTIFICATION

◆ This rhythm strip is from a 59-year-old woman who complained of sudden weakness in her legs and fell to the floor in her kitchen. Identify the rhythm (lead II).

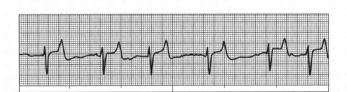

RHYTHM IDENTIFICATION

◆ This rhythm strip is from a 76-year-old man who was playing golf and experienced a syncopal episode. Identify the rhythm.

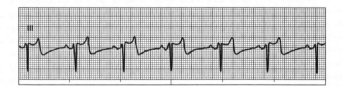

RHYTHM IDENTIFICATION

◆ This rhythm strip is from an 82-year-old woman with vomiting × 2 days. Identify the rhythm (lead II).

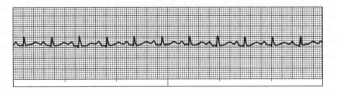

RHYTHM IDENTIFICATION

◆ These rhythm strips are from a 44-year-old woman complaining of chest pain. Identify the rhythm.

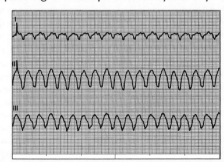

RHYTHM IDENTIFICATION

Narrow-QRS tachycardia (supraventricular tachycardia [SVT]) with ST-segment depression
- Ventricular rhythm ..... Regular
- Ventricular rate 167/min
- Atrial rhythm ..... Unable to determine
- Atrial rate ..... Unable to determine
- PRI: ..... Unable to determine
- QRS: ..... 0.06 second

RHYTHM IDENTIFICATION

Atrial fibrillation (with ST-segment elevation)
- Ventricular rhythm ..... Irregular
- Ventricular rate ..... 94 to 108/min
- Atrial rhythm ..... Unable to determine
- Atrial rate ..... Unable to determine
- PRI: ..... Unable to determine
- QRS: ..... 0.10 second

RHYTHM IDENTIFICATION

Sinus arrhythmia
- Ventricular rhythm ..... Irregular
- Ventricular rate ..... 68 to 88/min
- Atrial rhythm ..... Irregular
- Atrial rate ..... 68 to 88/min
- PRI: ..... 0.12 second
- QRS: ..... 0.08 second

RHYTHM IDENTIFICATION

Sinus bradycardia
- Ventricular rhythm ..... Regular
- Ventricular rate 48/min
- Atrial rhythm ..... Regular
- Atrial rate 48/min
- PRI: ..... 0.16 second
- QRS: ..... 0.08 second

RHYTHM IDENTIFICATION

Sinus rhythm with ST-segment elevation
- Ventricular rhythm ..... Regular
- Ventricular rate 65/min
- Atrial rhythm ..... Regular
- Atrial rate 65/min
- PRI: ..... 0.16 second
- QRS: ..... 0.08 second

RHYTHM IDENTIFICATION

Atrial fibrillation (controlled) with ST-segment elevation
- Ventricular rhythm ..... Irregular
- Ventricular rate ..... 50 to 79/min
- Atrial rhythm ..... Unable to determine
- Atrial rate ..... Unable to determine
- PRI: ..... Unable to determine
- QRS: ..... 0.12 second

RHYTHM IDENTIFICATION

Monomorphic ventricular tachycardia
- Ventricular rhythm ..... Regular
- Ventricular rate 176/min
- Atrial rhythm ..... None
- Atrial rate ..... None
- PRI: ..... None
- QRS: ..... 0.12 to 0.14 second

RHYTHM IDENTIFICATION

Sinus tachycardia
- Ventricular rhythm ..... Regular
- Ventricular rate 115/min
- Atrial rhythm ..... Regular
- Atrial rate 115/min
- PRI: ..... 0.18 second
- QRS: ..... 0.06 second

RHYTHM IDENTIFICATION

◆ Identify the rhythm (lead II).

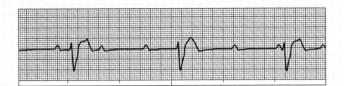

RHYTHM IDENTIFICATION

◆ Identify the rhythm (lead II).

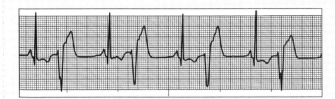

RHYTHM IDENTIFICATION

◆ This rhythm strip is from an 81-year-old woman complaining of chest pain. Identify the rhythm.

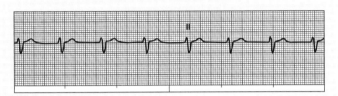

RHYTHM IDENTIFICATION

◆ Identify the rhythm (lead II).

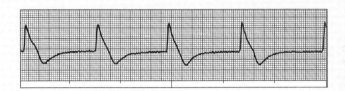

RHYTHM IDENTIFICATION

◆ This rhythm strip is from a 74-year-old woman complaining of weakness. Identify the rhythm (lead II).

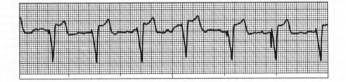

RHYTHM IDENTIFICATION

◆ These rhythm strips are from a 63-year-old woman who experienced a syncopal episode. Blood pressure 200/90. Blood sugar is 98. Identify the rhythm.

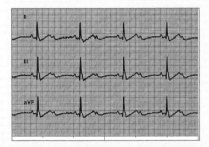

RHYTHM IDENTIFICATION

◆ Identify the rhythm (lead II).

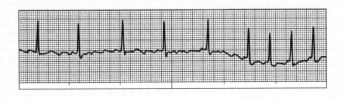

RHYTHM IDENTIFICATION

◆ This rhythm strip is from an 84-year-old woman with a nosebleed. Blood pressure 250/74. Identify the rhythm (lead II).

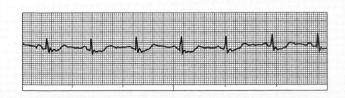

Sinus bradycardia with ventricular bigeminy
- ◆ Ventricular rhythm   Regular except for the event (every other beat is an ectopic beat)
- ◆ Ventricular rate   42/min (sinus beats)
- ◆ Atrial rhythm   Regular except for the event
- ◆ Atrial rate   42/min (sinus beats)
- ◆ PRI: 0.12 second (sinus beats)
- ◆ QRS: 0.08 to 0.10 second (sinus beats)

Complete (third-degree) AV block with ST-segment elevation
- ◆ Ventricular rhythm   Regular
- ◆ Ventricular rate   29/min
- ◆ Atrial rhythm   Regular
- ◆ Atrial rate   71/min
- ◆ PRI: Varies
- ◆ QRS: 0.16 second

Accelerated idioventricular rhythm (AIVR)
- ◆ Ventricular rhythm   Regular
- ◆ Ventricular rate   42/min
- ◆ Atrial rhythm   None
- ◆ Atrial rate   None
- ◆ PRI: None
- ◆ QRS: 0.24 second

Accelerated idioventricular rhythm (AIVR)
- ◆ Ventricular rhythm   Regular
- ◆ Ventricular rate   76/min
- ◆ Atrial rhythm   None
- ◆ Atrial rate   None
- ◆ PRI: None
- ◆ QRS: 0.12 to 0.14 second

Second-degree AV block, 2:1 conduction, probably type I
- ◆ Ventricular rhythm   Regular
- ◆ Ventricular rate   44/min
- ◆ Atrial rhythm   Regular
- ◆ Atrial rate   88/min
- ◆ PRI: 0.20 second
- ◆ QRS: 0.10 second

Ventricular demand pacemaker
- ◆ Atrial paced activity?   No
- ◆ Ventricular paced activity?   Yes
- ◆ Paced interval rate?   68

Sinus rhythm
- ◆ Ventricular rhythm   Regular
- ◆ Ventricular rate   68/min
- ◆ Atrial rhythm   Regular
- ◆ Atrial rate   68/min
- ◆ PRI: 0.16 second
- ◆ QRS: 0.08 second

Atrial flutter
- ◆ Ventricular rhythm   Irregular
- ◆ Ventricular rate   75 to 150/min
- ◆ Atrial rhythm   Unable to determine
- ◆ Atrial rate   Unable to determine
- ◆ PRI: Unable to determine
- ◆ QRS: 0.08 second

RHYTHM IDENTIFICATION

- This rhythm strip is from a 79-year-old man complaining of palpitations. His initial blood pressure was 112/84. His second blood pressure, 8 minutes after the first, was 78/P. Identify the rhythm (lead II).

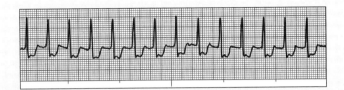

RHYTHM IDENTIFICATION

- This rhythm strip is from a 58-year-old man complaining of chest pain that he rates a 2 on a 1 to 10 scale. He states he recently began taking pills for weight control. Identify the rhythm (lead II).

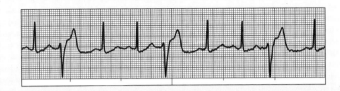

RHYTHM IDENTIFICATION

- Identify the rhythm.

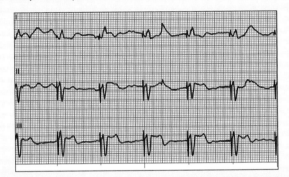

RHYTHM IDENTIFICATION

- This rhythm strip is from a 60-year-old woman complaining of palpitations and shortness of breath. Identify the rhythm.

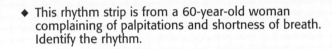

RHYTHM IDENTIFICATION

- This rhythm strip is from an 80-year-old man complaining of weakness and dizziness. Blood pressure 160/98. Blood sugar 88. Identify the rhythm (lead II).

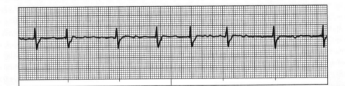

RHYTHM IDENTIFICATION

- This rhythm strip is from a 60-year-old woman complaining of palpitations and shortness of breath after administration of adenosine 6 mg IV. Identify the rhythm (lead II).

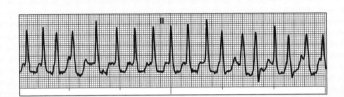

RHYTHM IDENTIFICATION

- Identify the rhythm (lead II).

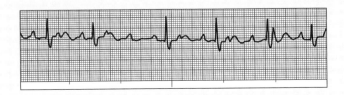

RHYTHM IDENTIFICATION

- This rhythm strip is from a 60-year-old woman complaining of palpitations and shortness of breath 2 minutes after administration of adenosine 6 mg IV. Identify the rhythm (lead II).

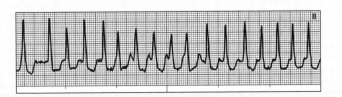

RHYTHM IDENTIFICATION

Sinus rhythm with uniform PVCs, ST-segment depression
- Ventricular rhythm   Regular except for the event(s)
- Ventricular rate   91/min (sinus beats)
- Atrial rhythm   Regular except for the event(s)
- Atrial rate   91/min (sinus beats)
- PRI: 0.20 second (sinus beats)
- QRS: 0.06 second (sinus beats)

RHYTHM IDENTIFICATION

Narrow-QRS tachycardia (supraventricular tachycardia [SVT]) with ST-segment depression
- Ventricular rhythm   Regular
- Ventricular rate   147/min
- Atrial rhythm   Unable to determine
- Atrial rate   Unable to determine
- PRI: Unable to determine
- QRS: 0.06 to 0.08 second

RHYTHM IDENTIFICATION

Atrial fibrillation with a rapid ventricular response
- Ventricular rhythm   Irregular
- Ventricular rate   130 to 214/min
- Atrial rhythm   Unable to determine
- Atrial rate   Unable to determine
- PRI: Unable to determine
- QRS: 0.08 second

RHYTHM IDENTIFICATION

100% ventricular paced rhythm
- Atrial paced activity?   No
- Ventricular paced activity?   Yes
- Paced interval rate?   60

RHYTHM IDENTIFICATION

Atrial fibrillation
- Ventricular rhythm   Irregular
- Ventricular rate   28 to 63/min
- Atrial rhythm   Unable to determine
- Atrial rate   Unable to determine
- PRI: Unable to determine
- QRS: 0.08 second

RHYTHM IDENTIFICATION

Atrial fibrillation (controlled)
- Ventricular rhythm   Irregular
- Ventricular rate   63 to 100/min
- Atrial rhythm   Unable to determine
- Atrial rate   Unable to determine
- PRI: Unable to determine
- QRS: 0.08 to 0.10 second

RHYTHM IDENTIFICATION

Atrial fibrillation with a rapid ventricular response
- Ventricular rhythm   Irregular
- Ventricular rate   115 to 250/min
- Atrial rhythm   Unable to determine
- Atrial rate   Unable to determine
- PRI: Unable to determine
- QRS: 0.08 second

RHYTHM IDENTIFICATION

Second-degree AV block type II
- Ventricular rhythm   Irregular
- Ventricular rate   42 to 71/min
- Atrial rhythm   Regular
- Atrial rate   125/min
- PRI: 0.24 second
- QRS: 0.10 to 0.12 second

RHYTHM IDENTIFICATION

◆ This rhythm strip is from a 60-year-old woman complaining of palpitations and shortness of breath 1 minute after administration of adenosine 12 mg IV. Identify the rhythm.

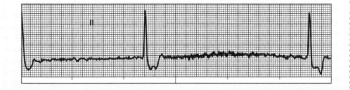

RHYTHM IDENTIFICATION

◆ Identify the rhythm (lead II).

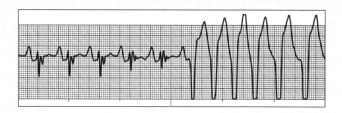

RHYTHM IDENTIFICATION

◆ Identify the rhythm (lead II).

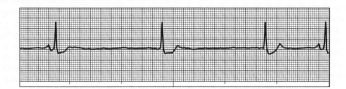

RHYTHM IDENTIFICATION

◆ Identify the rhythm (lead II).

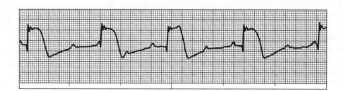

RHYTHM IDENTIFICATION

◆ This rhythm strip is from a 90-year-old woman with shortness of breath. Identify the rhythm (lead II).

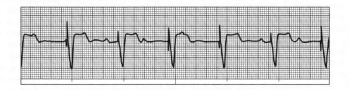

RHYTHM IDENTIFICATION

◆ Identify the rhythm (lead II).

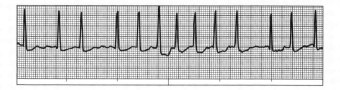

RHYTHM IDENTIFICATION

◆ Identify the rhythm (lead II).

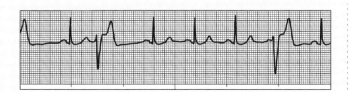

RHYTHM IDENTIFICATION

◆ Identify the rhythm (lead II).

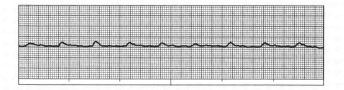

RHYTHM IDENTIFICATION

Sinus rhythm with first-degree AV block to monomorphic ventricular tachycardia (VT)
- Ventricular rhythm   Regular
- Ventricular rate   100/min (sinus beats) to 150/min (VT)
- Atrial rhythm   Regular to unable to determine
- Atrial rate   100/min (sinus beats)
- PRI: 0.24 second (sinus beats)
- QRS: 0.08 second (sinus beats)

RHYTHM IDENTIFICATION

Atrial fibrillation
- Ventricular rhythm   Irregular
- Ventricular rate   18 to 21/min
- Atrial rhythm   Unable to determine
- Atrial rate   Unable to determine
- PRI: Unable to determine
- QRS: 0.08 second

RHYTHM IDENTIFICATION

Complete (third-degree) AV block with ST-segment elevation
- Ventricular rhythm   Regular
- Ventricular rate   47/min
- Atrial rhythm   Regular
- Atrial rate   115/min
- PRI: Varies
- QRS: 0.08 second

RHYTHM IDENTIFICATION

Sinus beat, two junctional beats, sinus beat; ST-segment depression
- Ventricular rhythm   Irregular (sinus beats)
- Ventricular rate   0 to 70/min (sinus beats)
- Atrial rhythm   Irregular (sinus beats)
- Atrial rate   0 to 70/min (sinus beats)
- PRI: 0.16 second
- QRS: 0.06 second

RHYTHM IDENTIFICATION

Atrial fibrillation
- Ventricular rhythm   Irregular
- Ventricular rate   88 to 167/min
- Atrial rhythm   Unable to determine
- Atrial rate   Unable to determine
- PRI: Unable to determine
- QRS: 0.06 to 0.08 second

RHYTHM IDENTIFICATION

100% ventricular paced rhythm
- Atrial paced activity?   No
- Ventricular paced activity?   Yes
- Paced interval rate?   60

RHYTHM IDENTIFICATION

P-wave asystole
- Ventricular rhythm   None
- Ventricular rate   None
- Atrial rhythm   Regular
- Atrial rate   94/min
- PRI: None
- QRS: None

RHYTHM IDENTIFICATION

Sinus rhythm with uniform PVCs
- Ventricular rhythm   Regular except for the event(s)
- Ventricular rate   75/min (sinus beats)
- Atrial rhythm   Regular except for the event(s)
- Atrial rate   75/min (sinus beats)
- PRI: 0.16 to 0.18 second (sinus beats)
- QRS: 0.04 to 0.06 second (sinus beats)

RHYTHM IDENTIFICATION

◆ This rhythm strip is from a 74-year-old woman complaining of chest pain. Blood pressure 192/90. She rates her pain a 9 on a 1 to 10 scale. Identify the rhythm (lead II).

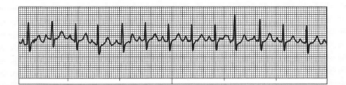

RHYTHM IDENTIFICATION

◆ This rhythm strip is from an 85-year-old woman with an altered level of responsiveness. Blood pressure 136/78. Blood sugar is 96. Identify the rhythm (lead II).

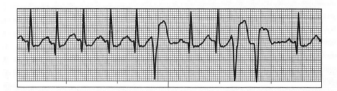

RHYTHM IDENTIFICATION

◆ Identify the rhythm (lead II).

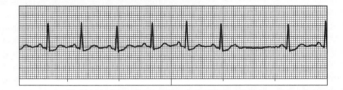

RHYTHM IDENTIFICATION

◆ This rhythm strip is from an 88-year-old man complaining of chest pain that he rates a 6 on a 1 to 10 scale. Blood pressure 170/80. Identify the rhythm (lead II).

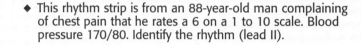
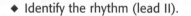
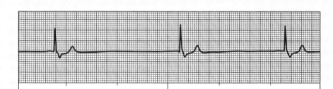

RHYTHM IDENTIFICATION

◆ Identify the rhythm (lead II).

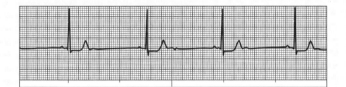

RHYTHM IDENTIFICATION

◆ Identify the rhythm (lead II).

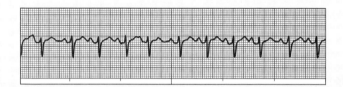

RHYTHM IDENTIFICATION

◆ This rhythm strip is from a 97-year-old man complaining of chest pain. Identify the rhythm (lead II).

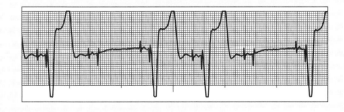

RHYTHM IDENTIFICATION

◆ Identify the rhythm.

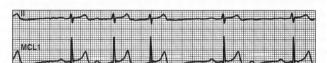

RHYTHM IDENTIFICATION

Sinus tachycardia with a PVC and a ventricular couplet
- ◆ Ventricular rhythm   Regular except for the event
- ◆ Ventricular rate   115/min (sinus beats)
- ◆ Atrial rhythm   Regular except for the event
- ◆ Atrial rate   115/min (sinus beats)
- ◆ PRI: 0.20 second (sinus beats)
- ◆ QRS: 0.08 to 0.10 second (sinus beats)

RHYTHM IDENTIFICATION

Sinus tachycardia
- ◆ Ventricular rhythm   Regular
- ◆ Ventricular rate   136/min
- ◆ Atrial rhythm   Regular
- ◆ Atrial rate   136/min
- ◆ PRI: 0.14 second
- ◆ QRS: 0.08 second

RHYTHM IDENTIFICATION

Sinus tachycardia with PACs
- ◆ Ventricular rhythm   Regular except for the event
- ◆ Ventricular rate   115/min (sinus beats)
- ◆ Atrial rhythm   Regular except for the event
- ◆ Atrial rate   115/min (sinus beats)
- ◆ PRI: 0.16 second
- ◆ QRS: 0.08 second

RHYTHM IDENTIFICATION

Sinus rhythm with a nonconducted PAC
- ◆ Ventricular rhythm   Regular except for the event
- ◆ Ventricular rate   91/min
- ◆ Atrial rhythm   Regular except for the event
- ◆ Atrial rate   91/min
- ◆ PRI: 0.16 second
- ◆ QRS: 0.06 second

RHYTHM IDENTIFICATION

Junctional bradycardia with ST-segment depression
- ◆ Ventricular rhythm   Essentially regular
- ◆ Ventricular rate   29/min
- ◆ Atrial rhythm   None
- ◆ Atrial rate   None
- ◆ PRI: None
- ◆ QRS: 0.04 to 0.06 second

RHYTHM IDENTIFICATION

Sinus bradycardia with ST-segment depression
- ◆ Ventricular rhythm   Regular
- ◆ Ventricular rate   35/min
- ◆ Atrial rhythm   Regular
- ◆ Atrial rate   35/min
- ◆ PRI: 0.16 second
- ◆ QRS: 0.06 second

Note: U waves are present (they follow the T waves).

RHYTHM IDENTIFICATION

Second-degree AV block type I
- ◆ Ventricular rhythm   Irregular
- ◆ Ventricular rate   42 to 81/min
- ◆ Atrial rhythm   Regular
- ◆ Atrial rate   75/min
- ◆ PRI: Lengthens
- ◆ QRS: 0.08 second

RHYTHM IDENTIFICATION

AV sequential pacemaker with failure to capture
- ◆ Atrial paced activity?   Yes
- ◆ Ventricular paced activity?   Yes
- ◆ Paced interval rate?   60

RHYTHM IDENTIFICATION

◆ Identify the rhythm (lead II).

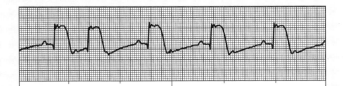

RHYTHM IDENTIFICATION

◆ This rhythm strip is from a 32-year-old woman who was sexually assaulted. Identify the rhythm (lead II).

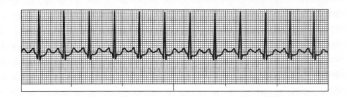

RHYTHM IDENTIFICATION

◆ These rhythm strips are from a 44-year-old man complaining of dizziness secondary to cocaine use. Identify the rhythm.

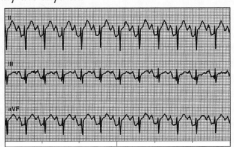

RHYTHM IDENTIFICATION

◆ These rhythm strips are from an 80-year-old woman after a fall injury. Identify the rhythm.

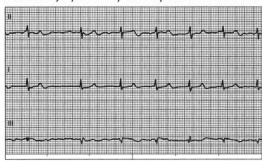

RHYTHM IDENTIFICATION

◆ Identify the rhythm (lead II).

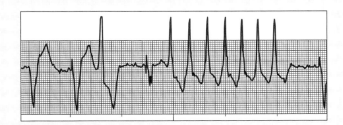

RHYTHM IDENTIFICATION

◆ Identify the rhythm (lead II).

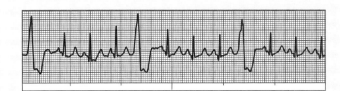

RHYTHM IDENTIFICATION

◆ Identify the rhythm (lead II).

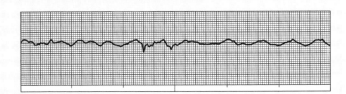

RHYTHM IDENTIFICATION

◆ This rhythm strip is from a 91-year-old woman who was found unresponsive. Healthcare professionals were unable to obtain a blood pressure, but her respiratory rate was 24/min. Identify the rhythm (lead II).

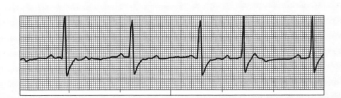

RHYTHM IDENTIFICATION

Sinus tachycardia
- ◆ Ventricular rhythm — Regular
- ◆ Ventricular rate — 122/min
- ◆ Atrial rhythm — Regular
- ◆ Atrial rate — 122/min
- ◆ PRI: — 0.16 second
- ◆ QRS: — 0.08 second

RHYTHM IDENTIFICATION

Second-degree AV block type 1 to 2:1 conduction, ST-segment elevation
- ◆ Ventricular rhythm — Irregular
- ◆ Ventricular rate — 48/min
- ◆ Atrial rhythm — Regular
- ◆ Atrial rate — 100/min
- ◆ PRI: — 0.24 second
- ◆ QRS: — 0.04 second

RHYTHM IDENTIFICATION

Atrial fibrillation (controlled) with ST-segment depression
- ◆ Ventricular rhythm — Irregular
- ◆ Ventricular rate — 47 to 79/min
- ◆ Atrial rhythm — Unable to determine
- ◆ Atrial rate — Unable to determine
- ◆ PRI: — Unable to determine
- ◆ QRS: — 0.06 to 0.08 second

RHYTHM IDENTIFICATION

Sinus tachycardia with ST-segment elevation
- ◆ Ventricular rhythm — Regular
- ◆ Ventricular rate — 115/min
- ◆ Atrial rhythm — Regular
- ◆ Atrial rate — 115/min
- ◆ PRI: — 0.20 second
- ◆ QRS: — 0.08 second

RHYTHM IDENTIFICATION

Sinus tachycardia with ventricular quadrigeminy
- ◆ Ventricular rhythm — Regular except for the event (every fourth beat is an ectopic beat)
- ◆ Ventricular rate — 115/min (sinus beats)
- ◆ Atrial rhythm — Regular except for the event
- ◆ Atrial rate — 115/min (sinus beats)
- ◆ PRI: — 0.12 second (sinus beats)
- ◆ QRS: — 0.06 second (sinus beats)

RHYTHM IDENTIFICATION

Ventricular paced rhythm with a PVC, a paced beat, nonsustained ventricular tachycardia, and a paced beat
- ◆ Atrial paced activity? — No
- ◆ Ventricular paced activity? — Yes
- ◆ Paced interval rate? — 71

RHYTHM IDENTIFICATION

Second-degree AV block type 1
- ◆ Ventricular rhythm — Irregular
- ◆ Ventricular rate — 45 to 94/min
- ◆ Atrial rhythm — Regular
- ◆ Atrial rate — 94/min
- ◆ PRI: — Lengthens
- ◆ QRS: — 0.10 second

RHYTHM IDENTIFICATION

Ventricular fibrillation
- ◆ Ventricular rhythm — Unable to determine
- ◆ Ventricular rate — Unable to determine
- ◆ Atrial rhythm — Unable to determine
- ◆ Atrial rate — Unable to determine
- ◆ PRI: — Unable to determine
- ◆ QRS: — Unable to determine

RHYTHM IDENTIFICATION

- This rhythm strip is from a 37-year-old woman complaining of shortness of breath and a fluttering sensation in her chest. Identify the rhythm (lead II).

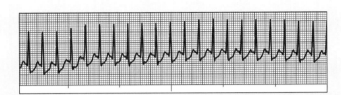

RHYTHM IDENTIFICATION

- Identify the rhythm (lead II).

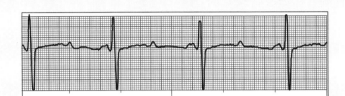

RHYTHM IDENTIFICATION

- This rhythm strip is from a 76-year-old woman complaining of weakness. Identify the rhythm.

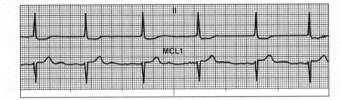

RHYTHM IDENTIFICATION

- This rhythm strip is from a 37-year-old asymptomatic man. Identify the rhythm.

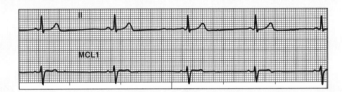

RHYTHM IDENTIFICATION

- This rhythm strip is from a 42-year-old man complaining of chest pain. Identify the rhythm (lead II).

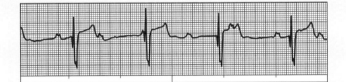

RHYTHM IDENTIFICATION

- This rhythm strip is from a 73-year-old woman complaining of dizziness and palpitations. Her blood pressure is 100/P. Identify the rhythm (lead II).

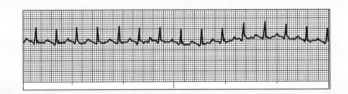

RHYTHM IDENTIFICATION

- This rhythm strip is from an 81-year-old man with weakness and an altered level of responsiveness. Identify the rhythm (lead II).

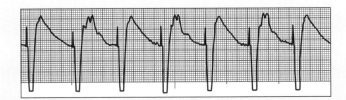

RHYTHM IDENTIFICATION

- This rhythm strip is from a 73-year-old woman complaining of dizziness and palpitations. Her blood pressure is 100/P. Identify the rhythm (lead II).

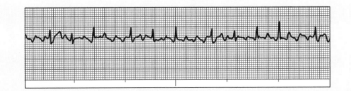

Second-degree AV block type II
- ◆ Ventricular rhythm   Regular
- ◆ Ventricular rate   37/min
- ◆ Atrial rhythm   Essentially regular
- ◆ Atrial rate   65/min
- ◆ PRI: 0.20 second
- ◆ QRS: 0.16 second

Narrow-QRS tachycardia (supraventricular tachycardia [SVT]) with ST-segment depression
- ◆ Ventricular rhythm   Regular
- ◆ Ventricular rate   214/min
- ◆ Atrial rhythm   Unable to determine
- ◆ Atrial rate   Unable to determine
- ◆ PRI: Unable to determine
- ◆ QRS: 0.06 to 0.08 second

Note: After a 6-mg IV dose of adenosine, and then a 12-mg dose, the patient converted to a sinus tachycardia at 110/min.

Sinus bradycardia
- ◆ Ventricular rhythm   Regular
- ◆ Ventricular rate   37/min
- ◆ Atrial rhythm   Regular
- ◆ Atrial rate   37/min
- ◆ PRI: 0.16 second
- ◆ QRS: 0.08 to 0.10 second

Junctional escape rhythm
- ◆ Ventricular rhythm   Regular
- ◆ Ventricular rate   57/min
- ◆ Atrial rhythm   None
- ◆ Atrial rate   None
- ◆ PRI: None
- ◆ QRS: 0.06 to 0.08 second

Atrial flutter
- ◆ Ventricular rhythm   Regular
- ◆ Ventricular rate   150/min
- ◆ Atrial rhythm   Unable to determine
- ◆ Atrial rate   Unable to determine
- ◆ PRI: Unable to determine
- ◆ QRS: 0.08 second

Complete (third-degree) AV block with ST-segment elevation
- ◆ Ventricular rhythm   Regular
- ◆ Ventricular rate   42/min
- ◆ Atrial rhythm   Regular
- ◆ Atrial rate   71/min
- ◆ PRI: Varies
- ◆ QRS: 0.12 second

Atrial flutter
- ◆ Ventricular rhythm   Irregular
- ◆ Ventricular rate   83 to 150/min
- ◆ Atrial rhythm   Unable to determine
- ◆ Atrial rate   Unable to determine
- ◆ PRI: Unable to determine
- ◆ QRS: 0.08 second

100% ventricular paced rhythm
- ◆ Atrial paced activity?   No
- ◆ Ventricular paced activity?   Yes
- ◆ Paced interval rate?   71

◆ A 76-year-old woman was found unresponsive, apneic, and pulseless. The following rhythm was observed after performing CPR and administration of IV epinephrine and atropine. Identify the rhythm.

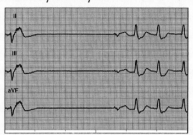

◆ Identify the rhythm (lead II).

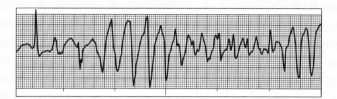

◆ Identify the rhythm (lead II).

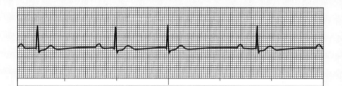

◆ Identify the rhythm.

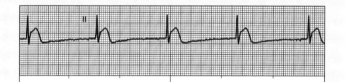

◆ Identify the rhythm (lead II).

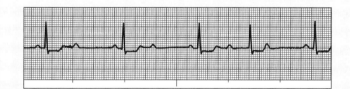

◆ This rhythm strip is from an 82-year-old man complaining of left leg pain. He states he has a permanent pacemaker. Blood pressure 128/84. Blood sugar is 241. Identify the rhythm (lead II).

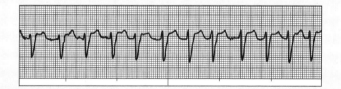

◆ Identify the rhythm (lead II).

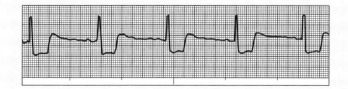

◆ This rhythm strip is from an 80-year-old woman complaining of chest pain. Her Blood pressure is 140/78. She states she had a new pacemaker "installed" 13 days ago. Identify the rhythm (lead II).

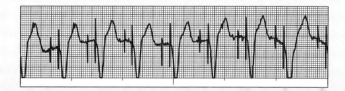

RHYTHM IDENTIFICATION

Polymorphic ventricular tachycardia
- Ventricular rhythm — Irregular
- Ventricular rate — 250 to 333/min
- Atrial rhythm — Unable to determine
- Atrial rate — Unable to determine
- PRI: — Unable to determine
- QRS: — 0.16 second

RHYTHM IDENTIFICATION

Agonal rhythm to sinus arrhythmia with a wide-QRS
- Ventricular rhythm — Irregular
- Ventricular rate — 68 to 75/min (sinus beats)
- Atrial rhythm — Irregular
- Atrial rate — 68 to 75/min (sinus beats)
- PRI: — 0.12 second
- QRS: — 0.10 to 0.12 second

RHYTHM IDENTIFICATION

Junctional escape rhythm
- Ventricular rhythm — Regular
- Ventricular rate — 44/min
- Atrial rhythm — Regular
- Atrial rate — 44/min
- PRI: — 0.14 second
- QRS: — 0.08 second

RHYTHM IDENTIFICATION

Sinus bradycardia with first-degree AV block and a PJC
- Ventricular rhythm — Regular except for the event
- Ventricular rate — 39/min
- Atrial rhythm — Regular except for the event
- Atrial rate — 39/min
- PRI: — 0.36 second
- QRS: — 0.06 second

RHYTHM IDENTIFICATION

Atrial fibrillation with a wide-QRS and ST-segment elevation
- Ventricular rhythm — Irregular
- Ventricular rate — 107 to 150/min
- Atrial rhythm — Unable to determine
- Atrial rate — Unable to determine
- PRI: — Unable to determine
- QRS: — 0.12 second

RHYTHM IDENTIFICATION

Second-degree AV block type I with ST-segment depression
- Ventricular rhythm — Irregular
- Ventricular rate — 41 to 63/min
- Atrial rhythm — Regular
- Atrial rate — 88/min
- PRI: — Lengthens
- QRS: — 0.08 to 0.10 second

RHYTHM IDENTIFICATION

100% paced rhythm—AV sequential pacemaker
- Atrial paced activity? — Yes
- Ventricular paced activity? — Yes
- Paced interval rate? — 83

RHYTHM IDENTIFICATION

Sinus bradycardia with ST-segment depression
- Ventricular rhythm — Regular
- Ventricular rate — 44/min
- Atrial rhythm — Regular
- Atrial rate — 44/min
- PRI: — 0.20 second
- QRS: — 0.06 second

RHYTHM IDENTIFICATION

◆ Identify the rhythm (lead II).

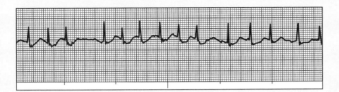

RHYTHM IDENTIFICATION

◆ These rhythm strips are from a 72-year-old man complaining of feeling weak and tired. Identify the rhythm.

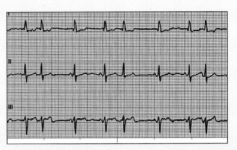

RHYTHM IDENTIFICATION

◆ Identify the rhythm (lead II).

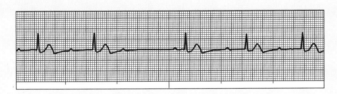

RHYTHM IDENTIFICATION

◆ This rhythm strip is from a 39-year-old man complaining of "feeling faint." Blood pressure 200/120. Identify the rhythm (lead II).

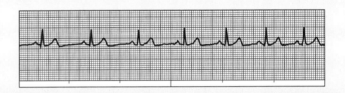

RHYTHM IDENTIFICATION

◆ Identify the rhythm (lead II).

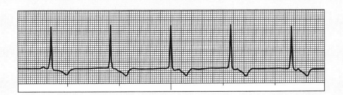

RHYTHM IDENTIFICATION

◆ This rhythm strip is from an 87-year-old woman with an altered level of responsiveness. Identify the rhythm (lead II).

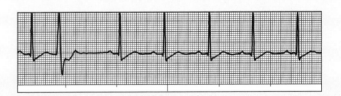

RHYTHM IDENTIFICATION

◆ This rhythm strip is from a 50-year-old man complaining of chest pressure. Blood pressure 70/50. Identify the rhythm (lead II).

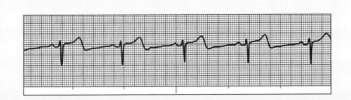

RHYTHM IDENTIFICATION

◆ Identify the rhythm (lead II).

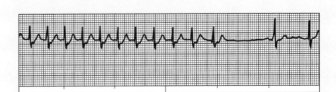

RHYTHM IDENTIFICATION

Sinus rhythm with PACs
- ◆ Ventricular rhythm — Regular except for the event
- ◆ Ventricular rate — 75/min (sinus beats)
- ◆ Atrial rhythm — Regular except for the event
- ◆ Atrial rate — 75/min (sinus beats)
- ◆ PRI: — 0.12 to 0.14 second
- ◆ QRS: — 0.06 second

RHYTHM IDENTIFICATION

Atrial fibrillation (uncontrolled) with ST-segment depression
- ◆ Ventricular rhythm — Irregular
- ◆ Ventricular rate — 83 to 167/min
- ◆ Atrial rhythm — Unable to determine
- ◆ Atrial rate — Unable to determine
- ◆ PRI: — Unable to determine
- ◆ QRS: — 0.08 second

RHYTHM IDENTIFICATION

Sinus arrhythmia
- ◆ Ventricular rhythm — Irregular
- ◆ Ventricular rate — 67 to 83/min
- ◆ Atrial rhythm — Irregular
- ◆ Atrial rate — 67 to 83/min
- ◆ PRI: — 0.16 second
- ◆ QRS: — 0.06 to 0.08 second

RHYTHM IDENTIFICATION

Second-degree AV block type I
- ◆ Ventricular rhythm — Irregular
- ◆ Ventricular rate — 34 to 52/min
- ◆ Atrial rhythm — Regular
- ◆ Atrial rate — 60/min
- ◆ PRI: — Lengthens
- ◆ QRS: — 0.06 to 0.08 second

RHYTHM IDENTIFICATION

Sinus rhythm with first-degree AV block and a PVC
- ◆ Ventricular rhythm — Regular except for the event
- ◆ Ventricular rate — 71/min (sinus beats)
- ◆ Atrial rhythm — Regular except for the event
- ◆ Atrial rate — 71/min (sinus beats)
- ◆ PRI: — 0.22 second (sinus beats)
- ◆ QRS: — 0.10 second (sinus beats)

RHYTHM IDENTIFICATION

Sinus beat to junctional escape rhythm with inverted T waves
- ◆ Ventricular rhythm — Regular
- ◆ Ventricular rate — 52/min
- ◆ Atrial rhythm — None
- ◆ Atrial rate — None
- ◆ PRI: — None
- ◆ QRS: — 0.06 second

RHYTHM IDENTIFICATION

Conversion from narrow-QRS tachycardia to sinus rhythm with a first-degree AV block
- ◆ Ventricular rhythm — Regular (sinus beats)
- ◆ Ventricular rate — 88/min (sinus beats)
- ◆ Atrial rhythm — Regular (sinus beats)
- ◆ Atrial rate — 88/min (sinus beats)
- ◆ PRI: — 0.22 second (sinus beats)
- ◆ QRS: — 0.08 second (sinus beats)

RHYTHM IDENTIFICATION

Sinus bradycardia with ST-segment elevation
- ◆ Ventricular rhythm — Regular
- ◆ Ventricular rate — 52/min
- ◆ Atrial rhythm — Regular
- ◆ Atrial rate — 52/min
- ◆ PRI: — 0.18 to 0.20 second
- ◆ QRS: — 0.10 second

◆ Identify the rhythm (lead II).

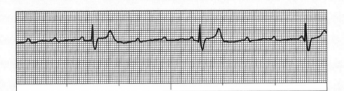

◆ Identify the rhythm (lead II).

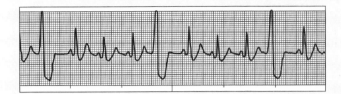

◆ Identify the rhythm.

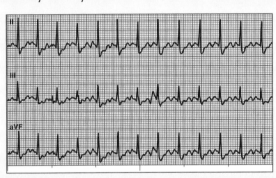

◆ This rhythm strip is from a 32-year-old woman complaining of dizziness and shortness of breath. Identify the rhythm (lead II).

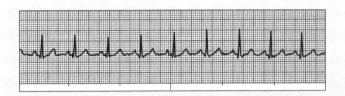

◆ Identify the rhythm (lead II).

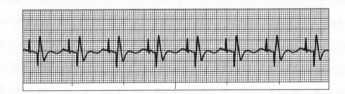

◆ This rhythm strip is from a 79-year-old man who experienced a syncopal episode. He has a history of seizures. Identify the rhythm (lead II).

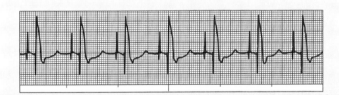

◆ Identify the rhythm (lead II).

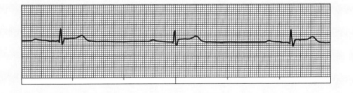

◆ Identify the rhythm (lead II).

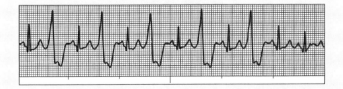

Sinus tachycardia with ventricular quadrigeminy, ST-segment depression

- ◆ Ventricular rhythm — Regular except for the event (every fourth beat is an ectopic beat)
- ◆ Ventricular rate — 107/min (sinus beats)
- ◆ Atrial rhythm — Regular except for the event
- ◆ Atrial rate — 107/min (sinus beats)
- ◆ PRI: — 0.12 second (sinus beats)
- ◆ QRS: — 0.06 second (sinus beats)

Complete (third-degree) AV block

- ◆ Ventricular rhythm — Regular
- ◆ Ventricular rate — 29/min
- ◆ Atrial rhythm — Regular
- ◆ Atrial rate — 115/min
- ◆ PRI: — Varies
- ◆ QRS: — 0.08 second

Sinus rhythm

- ◆ Ventricular rhythm — Regular
- ◆ Ventricular rate — 94/min
- ◆ Atrial rhythm — Regular
- ◆ Atrial rate — 94/min
- ◆ PRI: — 0.16 second
- ◆ QRS: — 0.06 second

Atrial flutter with ST-segment depression

- ◆ Ventricular rhythm — Regular
- ◆ Ventricular rate — 128/min
- ◆ Atrial rhythm — Unable to determine
- ◆ Atrial rate — Unable to determine
- ◆ PRI: — Unable to determine
- ◆ QRS: — 0.06 to 0.08 second

100% paced rhythm—AV sequential pacemaker

- ◆ Atrial paced activity? — Yes
- ◆ Ventricular paced activity? — Yes
- ◆ Paced interval rate? — 70

100% paced rhythm—AV sequential pacemaker

- ◆ Atrial paced activity? — Yes
- ◆ Ventricular paced activity? — Yes
- ◆ Paced interval rate? — 79

Sinus tachycardia with frequent uniform PVCs

- ◆ Ventricular rhythm — Irregular
- ◆ Ventricular rate — 120/min (sinus beats)
- ◆ Atrial rhythm — Irregular
- ◆ Atrial rate — 120/min (sinus beats)
- ◆ PRI: — 0.12 second (sinus beats)
- ◆ QRS: — 0.08 second (sinus beats)

Sinus bradycardia with first-degree AV block, ST-segment elevation

- ◆ Ventricular rhythm — Regular
- ◆ Ventricular rate — 23/min
- ◆ Atrial rhythm — Regular
- ◆ Atrial rate — 23/min
- ◆ PRI: — 0.44 second
- ◆ QRS: — 0.08 second

RHYTHM IDENTIFICATION

◆ Identify the rhythm (lead II).

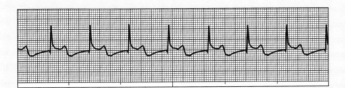

RHYTHM IDENTIFICATION

◆ This rhythm strip is from a 61-year-old woman with an altered level of responsiveness. Blood pressure 112/62. Blood sugar is 42. Identify the rhythm (lead II).

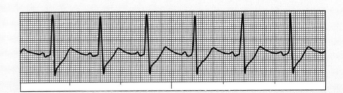

RHYTHM IDENTIFICATION

◆ This rhythm strip is from an 88-year-old woman complaining of dizziness. Blood pressure 176/68. Identify the rhythm (lead II).

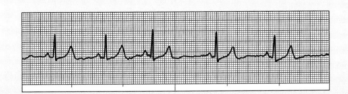

RHYTHM IDENTIFICATION

◆ This rhythm strip is from a 61-year-old woman complaining of shortness of breath. Blood pressure 176/110. Identify the rhythm (lead II).

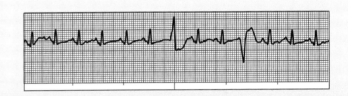

RHYTHM IDENTIFICATION

◆ These rhythm strips are from a 52-year-old man with syncope. Identify the rhythm.

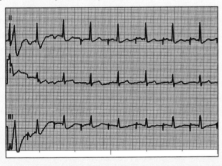

RHYTHM IDENTIFICATION

◆ Identify the rhythm.

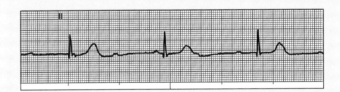

RHYTHM IDENTIFICATION

◆ Identify the rhythm.

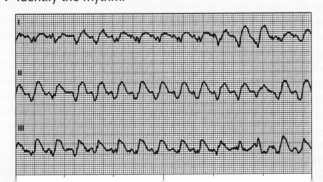

RHYTHM IDENTIFICATION

◆ This rhythm strip is from an 85-year-old woman complaining of weakness. Identify the rhythm.

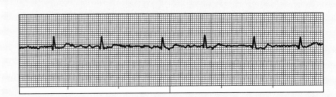

RHYTHM IDENTIFICATION

Sinus rhythm with ST-segment depression
- ◆ Ventricular rhythm   Regular
- ◆ Ventricular rate   65/min
- ◆ Atrial rhythm   Regular
- ◆ Atrial rate   65/min
- ◆ PRI: 0.20 second
- ◆ QRS: 0.10 second

RHYTHM IDENTIFICATION

Accelerated junctional rhythm with ST-segment elevation
- ◆ Ventricular rhythm   Regular
- ◆ Ventricular rate   79/min
- ◆ Atrial rhythm   None
- ◆ Atrial rate   None
- ◆ PRI: None
- ◆ QRS: 0.08 second

RHYTHM IDENTIFICATION

Sinus tachycardia with multiform PVCs
- ◆ Ventricular rhythm   Essentially regular except for the events
- ◆ Ventricular rate   125/min
- ◆ Atrial rhythm   Essentially regular except for the events
- ◆ Atrial rate   125/min
- ◆ PRI: 0.12 second (sinus beats)
- ◆ QRS: 0.06 second (sinus beats)

RHYTHM IDENTIFICATION

Sinus rhythm with a PAC
- ◆ Ventricular rhythm   Regular except for the event
- ◆ Ventricular rate   60/min (sinus beats)
- ◆ Atrial rhythm   Regular except for the event
- ◆ Atrial rate   60/min (sinus beats)
- ◆ PRI: 0.16 second
- ◆ QRS: 0.08 second

RHYTHM IDENTIFICATION

Complete (third-degree) AV block
- ◆ Ventricular rhythm   Regular
- ◆ Ventricular rate   32/min
- ◆ Atrial rhythm   Regular
- ◆ Atrial rate   79/min
- ◆ PRI: Varies
- ◆ QRS: 0.12 second

RHYTHM IDENTIFICATION

Atrial pacemaker
- ◆ Atrial paced activity?   Yes
- ◆ Ventricular paced activity?   No
- ◆ Paced interval rate?   79

RHYTHM IDENTIFICATION

Atrial fibrillation (controlled)
- ◆ Ventricular rhythm   Irregular
- ◆ Ventricular rate   50 to 73/min
- ◆ Atrial rhythm   Unable to determine
- ◆ Atrial rate   Unable to determine
- ◆ PRI: Unable to determine
- ◆ QRS: 0.08 second

RHYTHM IDENTIFICATION

Monomorphic ventricular tachycardia
- ◆ Ventricular rhythm   Essentially regular
- ◆ Ventricular rate   150/min
- ◆ Atrial rhythm   Unable to determine
- ◆ Atrial rate   Unable to determine
- ◆ PRI: Unable to determine
- ◆ QRS: 0.12 to 0.16 second

RHYTHM IDENTIFICATION

- This rhythm strip is from an 87-year-old man complaining of chest pain. Identify the rhythm (lead II).

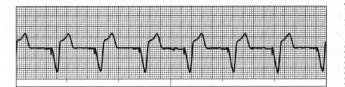

RHYTHM IDENTIFICATION

- This rhythm strip is from a 3-month-old infant. Identify the rhythm (lead II).

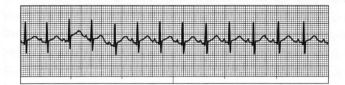

RHYTHM IDENTIFICATION

- Identify the rhythm (lead III).

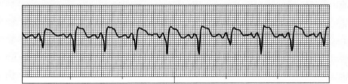

RHYTHM IDENTIFICATION

- Identify the rhythm (lead II).

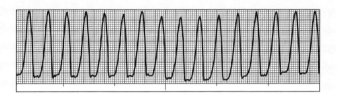

RHYTHM IDENTIFICATION

- This rhythm strip is from an 89-year-old woman complaining of weakness. She has a history of hypertension. Identify the rhythm (lead II).

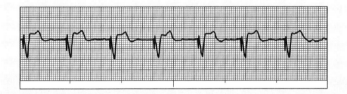

RHYTHM IDENTIFICATION

- Identify the rhythm (lead II).

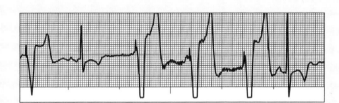

RHYTHM IDENTIFICATION

- This rhythm strip is from a 72-year-old man who presented with left-sided weakness. He had a history of a brain tumor. Identify the rhythm.

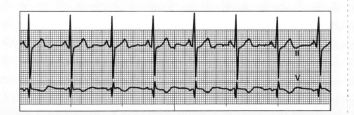

RHYTHM IDENTIFICATION

- This rhythm strip is from a 62-year-old woman who experienced a syncopal episode. Identify the rhythm (lead II).

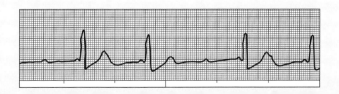

Sinus tachycardia
- Ventricular rhythm   Regular
- Ventricular rate   136/min
- Atrial rhythm   Regular
- Atrial rate   136/min
- PRI: 0.12 second
- QRS: 0.08 to 0.10 second

100% ventricular paced rhythm
- Atrial paced activity?   No
- Ventricular paced activity?   Yes
- Paced interval rate?   72

Monomorphic ventricular tachycardia
- Ventricular rhythm   Regular
- Ventricular rate   167/min
- Atrial rhythm   Unable to determine
- Atrial rate   Unable to determine
- PRI: Unable to determine
- QRS: 0.16 second

Accelerated junctional rhythm with ST-segment elevation
- Ventricular rhythm   Regular
- Ventricular rate   98/min
- Atrial rhythm   Regular
- Atrial rate   98/min
- PRI: 0.12 second
- QRS: 0.08 second

Sinus rhythm with a ventricular demand pacer
- Atrial paced activity?   No
- Ventricular paced activity?   Yes
- Paced interval rate?   57

100% ventricular paced rhythm
- Atrial paced activity?   No
- Ventricular paced activity?   Yes
- Paced interval rate?   72

Second-degree AV block type II
- Ventricular rhythm   Irregular
- Ventricular rate   33 to 47/min
- Atrial rhythm   Regular
- Atrial rate   100/min
- PRI: 0.12 second
- QRS: 0.06 to 0.10 second

Sinus rhythm
- Ventricular rhythm   Regular
- Ventricular rate   75/min
- Atrial rhythm   Regular
- Atrial rate   75/min
- PRI: 0.12 second
- QRS: 0.08 second

RHYTHM IDENTIFICATION

◆ Identify the rhythm.

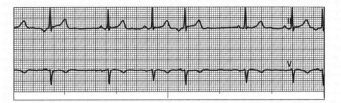

RHYTHM IDENTIFICATION

◆ Identify the rhythm (lead II).

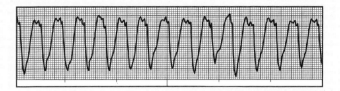

RHYTHM IDENTIFICATION

◆ This rhythm strip is from a 25-year-old asymptomatic paramedic student. Identify the rhythm (lead II).

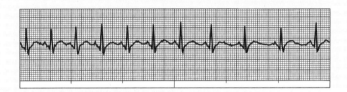

RHYTHM IDENTIFICATION

◆ Identify the rhythm.

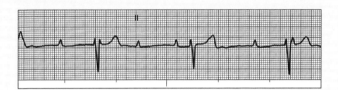

RHYTHM IDENTIFICATION

◆ This rhythm strip is from a 77-year-old man complaining of chest pain. His chest hit the steering wheel during a motor vehicle crash. Identify the rhythm (lead II).

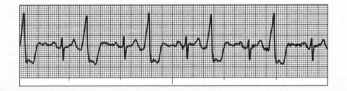

RHYTHM IDENTIFICATION

◆ Identify the rhythm (lead II).

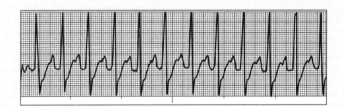

RHYTHM IDENTIFICATION

◆ This rhythm strip is from a 70-year-old woman complaining of chest pain. Identify the rhythm.

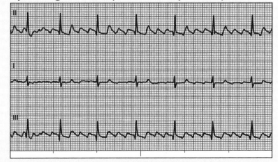

RHYTHM IDENTIFICATION

◆ Identify the rhythm (lead II).

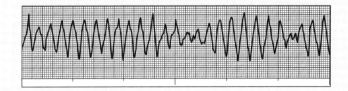

Monomorphic ventricular tachycardia
- Ventricular rhythm   Essentially regular
- Ventricular rate   150/min
- Atrial rhythm   Unable to determine
- Atrial rate   Unable to determine
- PRI: Unable to determine
- QRS: 0.24 second

Sinus rhythm with PJCs
- Ventricular rhythm   Regular except for the event (every third beat is a PJC)
- Ventricular rate   63/min (sinus beats)
- Atrial rhythm   Regular except for the event (every third beat is a PJC)
- Atrial rate   63/min (sinus beats)
- PRI: 0.12 to 0.16 second (sinus beats)
- QRS: 0.06 second (sinus beats)

Complete (third-degree) AV block
- Ventricular rhythm   Regular
- Ventricular rate   32/min
- Atrial rhythm   Regular
- Atrial rate   83/min
- PRI: Varies
- QRS: 0.10 to 0.12 second

Sinus tachyarrhythmia
- Ventricular rhythm   Irregular
- Ventricular rate   86 to 130/min
- Atrial rhythm   Irregular
- Atrial rate   86 to 130/min
- PRI: 0.12 second
- QRS: 0.08 to 0.10 second

Sinus tachycardia with ST-segment depression
- Ventricular rhythm   Regular
- Ventricular rate   116/min
- Atrial rhythm   Regular
- Atrial rate   116/min
- PRI: 0.20 second
- QRS: 0.10 second

Sinus bradycardia with ventricular bigeminy
- Ventricular rhythm   Regular except for the event (every other beat is an ectopic beat)
- Ventricular rate   52/min (sinus beats)
- Atrial rhythm   Regular except for the event
- Atrial rate   52/min (sinus beats)
- PRI: 0.16 second (sinus beats)
- QRS: 0.08 to 0.10 second (sinus beats)

Polymorphic ventricular tachycardia
- Ventricular rhythm   Irregular
- Ventricular rate   250 to 333/min
- Atrial rhythm   Unable to determine
- Atrial rate   Unable to determine
- PRI: Unable to determine
- QRS: 0.16 second

Atrial flutter
- Ventricular rhythm   Regular
- Ventricular rate   81/min
- Atrial rhythm   Unable to determine
- Atrial rate   Unable to determine
- PRI: Unable to determine
- QRS: 0.06 second

RHYTHM IDENTIFICATION

◆ Identify the rhythm.

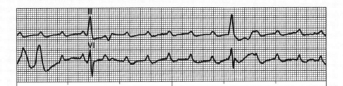

RHYTHM IDENTIFICATION

◆ This rhythm strip is from a 37-year-old woman complaining of palpitations. Identify the rhythm (lead II).

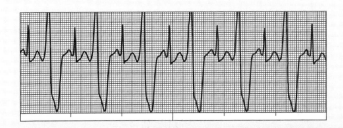

RHYTHM IDENTIFICATION

◆ This rhythm strip is from a 20-year-old man immediately after a seizure. Identify the rhythm (lead II).

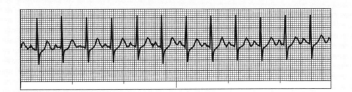

RHYTHM IDENTIFICATION

◆ This rhythm strip is from an 82-year-old man with an altered level of responsiveness. Although a weak pulse is present, a blood pressure is not palpable. His skin is cool, pale, and moist. Identify the rhythm (lead II).

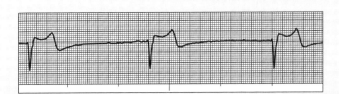

RHYTHM IDENTIFICATION

◆ This rhythm strip is from an 87-year-old man complaining of chest pain. Identify the rhythm (lead II).

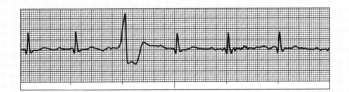

RHYTHM IDENTIFICATION

◆ Identify the rhythm.

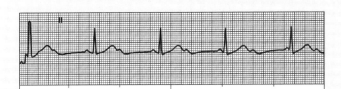

RHYTHM IDENTIFICATION

◆ Identify the rhythm (lead II).

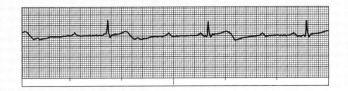

RHYTHM IDENTIFICATION

◆ This rhythm strip is from a 53-year-old man complaining of chest pressure and shortness of breath. Blood pressure is 130/86, respirations 20. He has a history of a spinal cord injury and coronary artery disease. Identify the rhythm (lead II).

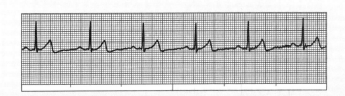

RHYTHM IDENTIFICATION

Sinus rhythm with ventricular bigeminy
- Ventricular rhythm   Regular except for the event (every other beat is an ectopic beat)
- Ventricular rate   65/min (sinus beats)
- Atrial rhythm   Regular except for the event
- Atrial rate   65/min (sinus beats)
- PRI: 0.16 second (sinus beats)
- QRS: 0.08 to 0.10 second (sinus beats)

RHYTHM IDENTIFICATION

Complete (third-degree) AV block with ST-segment depression
- Ventricular rhythm   Regular
- Ventricular rate   22/min
- Atrial rhythm   Regular
- Atrial rate   136/min
- PRI: Varies
- QRS: 0.12 to 0.14 second

RHYTHM IDENTIFICATION

Idioventricular (ventricular escape) rhythm
- Ventricular rhythm   Regular
- Ventricular rate   25/min
- Atrial rhythm   Unable to determine
- Atrial rate   Unable to determine
- PRI: Unable to determine
- QRS: 0.12 second

RHYTHM IDENTIFICATION

Sinus tachycardia
- Ventricular rhythm   Regular
- Ventricular rate   125/min
- Atrial rhythm   Regular
- Atrial rate   125/min
- PRI: 0.12 to 0.16 second
- QRS: 0.08 to 0.10 second

RHYTHM IDENTIFICATION

Second-degree AV block, 2:1 conduction, probably type I
- Ventricular rhythm   Regular
- Ventricular rate   46/min
- Atrial rhythm   Regular
- Atrial rate   92/min
- PRI: 0.12 second
- QRS: 0.08 second

RHYTHM IDENTIFICATION

Sinus rhythm with first-degree AV block and a PVC
- Ventricular rhythm   Regular except for the event
- Ventricular rate   60/min (sinus beats)
- Atrial rhythm   Regular except for the event
- Atrial rate   60/min (sinus beats)
- PRI: 0.32 second
- QRS: 0.10 second

RHYTHM IDENTIFICATION

Sinus bradycardia
- Ventricular rhythm   Regular
- Ventricular rate   58/min
- Atrial rhythm   Regular
- Atrial rate   58/min
- PRI: 0.20 second
- QRS: 0.06 second

RHYTHM IDENTIFICATION

Complete (third-degree) AV block
- Ventricular rhythm   Regular
- Ventricular rate   31/min
- Atrial rhythm   Regular
- Atrial rate   100/min
- PRI: Varies
- QRS: 0.06 second

RHYTHM IDENTIFICATION

- This rhythm strip is from a 67-year-old man complaining of dizziness. Blood pressure 182/100. Blood sugar is 134. Identify the rhythm (lead II).

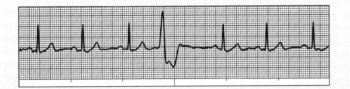

RHYTHM IDENTIFICATION

- This rhythm strip is from a 80-year-old woman who is complaining that "the room is spinning." Blood pressure 180/90. Identify the rhythm (lead II).

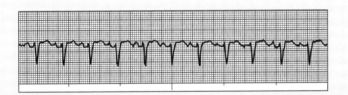

RHYTHM IDENTIFICATION

- Identify the rhythm (lead II).

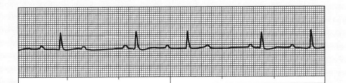

RHYTHM IDENTIFICATION

- This rhythm strip is from a 22-year-old woman complaining of abdominal pain. Blood pressure 140/78. Identify the rhythm (lead II).

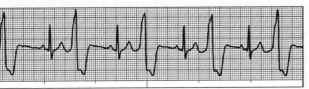

RHYTHM IDENTIFICATION

- Identify the rhythm.

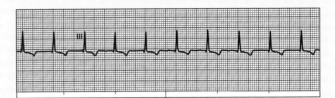

RHYTHM IDENTIFICATION

- Identify the rhythm (lead II).

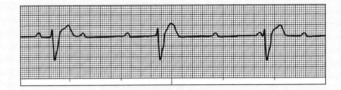

RHYTHM IDENTIFICATION

- Identify the rhythm (lead II).

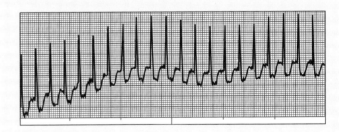

RHYTHM IDENTIFICATION

- This rhythm strip is from a 73-year-old woman complaining of chest pain. Identify the rhythm (lead II).

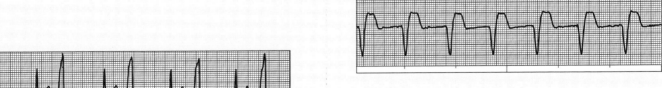

RHYTHM IDENTIFICATION

Accelerated junctional rhythm
- Ventricular rhythm   Regular
- Ventricular rate   100/min
- Atrial rhythm   None
- Atrial rate   None
- PRI: None
- QRS: 0.08 second

RHYTHM IDENTIFICATION

Sinus rhythm with a PVC
- Ventricular rhythm   Regular except for the event
- Ventricular rate   68/min (sinus beats)
- Atrial rhythm   Regular except for the event
- Atrial rate   68/min (sinus beats)
- PRI: 0.16 to 0.18 second (sinus beats)
- QRS: 0.06 second (sinus beats)

RHYTHM IDENTIFICATION

Complete (third-degree) AV block with ST-segment elevation
- Ventricular rhythm   Regular
- Ventricular rate   29/min
- Atrial rhythm   Regular
- Atrial rate   94/min
- PRI: Varies
- QRS: 0.16 second

RHYTHM IDENTIFICATION

Sinus tachycardia with a wide-QRS and ST-segment elevation
- Ventricular rhythm   Regular
- Ventricular rate   107/min
- Atrial rhythm   Regular
- Atrial rate   107/min
- PRI: 0.16 second
- QRS: 0.12 second

RHYTHM IDENTIFICATION

Narrow-QRS tachycardia with ST-segment depression
- Ventricular rhythm   Regular
- Ventricular rate   214/min
- Atrial rhythm   Unable to determine
- Atrial rate   Unable to determine
- PRI: Unable to determine
- QRS: 0.04 to 0.06 second

RHYTHM IDENTIFICATION

Second-degree AV block type I
- Ventricular rhythm   Irregular
- Ventricular rate   42 to 75/min
- Atrial rhythm   Regular
- Atrial rate   75/min
- PRI: Lengthens
- QRS: 0.06 second

RHYTHM IDENTIFICATION

Accelerated idioventricular rhythm (AIVR) with ST-segment elevation
- Ventricular rhythm   Regular
- Ventricular rate   71/min
- Atrial rhythm   Unable to determine
- Atrial rate   Unable to determine
- PRI: Unable to determine
- QRS: 0.12 second

RHYTHM IDENTIFICATION

Sinus bradycardia with ventricular bigeminy
- Ventricular rhythm   Regular except for the event (every other beat is an ectopic beat)
- Ventricular rate   43/min (sinus beats)
- Atrial rhythm   Regular except for the event
- Atrial rate   43/min (sinus beats)
- PRI: 0.16 second (sinus beats)
- QRS: 0.08 second (sinus beats)

RHYTHM IDENTIFICATION

◆ This rhythm strip is from an 18-year-old man with a gunshot wound to his chest. Identify the rhythm (lead II).

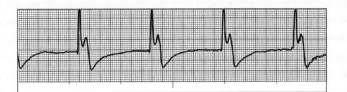

RHYTHM IDENTIFICATION

◆ This rhythm strip is from an 18-year-old male with a gunshot wound to his chest. Identify the rhythm (lead II).

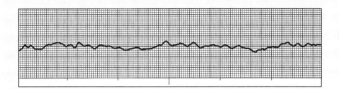

RHYTHM IDENTIFICATION

◆ This rhythm strip is from a 62-year-old man complaining of chest pain. Blood pressure 124/78. Identify the rhythm (lead II).

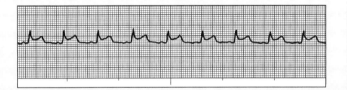

RHYTHM IDENTIFICATION

◆ This rhythm strip is from an 81-year-old woman complaining of shortness of breath. Her blood pressure is 162/74, respirations 20. Lung sounds are clear bilaterally. Identify the rhythm (lead II).

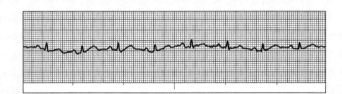

RHYTHM IDENTIFICATION

◆ Identify the rhythm (lead II).

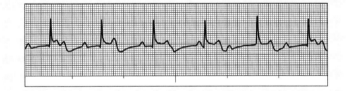

RHYTHM IDENTIFICATION

◆ This rhythm strip is from a 72-year-old man being transported for permanent pacemaker insertion. Identify the rhythm.

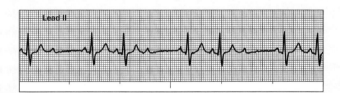

RHYTHM IDENTIFICATION

◆ Identify the rhythm.

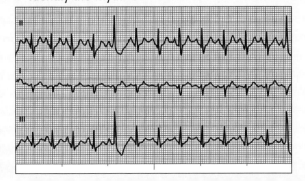

RHYTHM IDENTIFICATION

◆ Identify the rhythm.

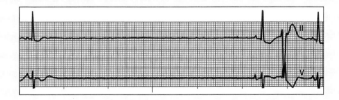

RHYTHM IDENTIFICATION

Ventricular fibrillation
- ◆ Ventricular rhythm   Unable to determine
- ◆ Ventricular rate   Unable to determine
- ◆ Atrial rhythm   Unable to determine
- ◆ Atrial rate   Unable to determine
- ◆ PRI: Unable to determine
- ◆ QRS: Unable to determine

RHYTHM IDENTIFICATION

Junctional escape rhythm with ST-segment elevation
- ◆ Ventricular rhythm   Regular
- ◆ Ventricular rate   44/min
- ◆ Atrial rhythm   None
- ◆ Atrial rate   None
- ◆ PRI: None
- ◆ QRS: 0.08 second

RHYTHM IDENTIFICATION

Sinus rhythm
- ◆ Ventricular rhythm   Regular
- ◆ Ventricular rate   86/min
- ◆ Atrial rhythm   Regular
- ◆ Atrial rate   86/min
- ◆ PRI: 0.18 to 0.20 second
- ◆ QRS: 0.06 second

RHYTHM IDENTIFICATION

Sinus rhythm with ST-segment elevation
- ◆ Ventricular rhythm   Regular
- ◆ Ventricular rate   93/min
- ◆ Atrial rhythm   Regular
- ◆ Atrial rate   93/min
- ◆ PRI: 0.14 second
- ◆ QRS: 0.08 second

RHYTHM IDENTIFICATION

Second-degree AV block type II
- ◆ Ventricular rhythm   Irregular
- ◆ Ventricular rate   48 to 94/min
- ◆ Atrial rhythm   Regular
- ◆ Atrial rate   94/min
- ◆ PRI: 0.16 second
- ◆ QRS: 0.12 second

RHYTHM IDENTIFICATION

Complete (third-degree) AV block with ST-segment elevation
- ◆ Ventricular rhythm   Regular
- ◆ Ventricular rate   58/min
- ◆ Atrial rhythm   Regular
- ◆ Atrial rate   100/min
- ◆ PRI: Varies
- ◆ QRS: 0.04 to 0.06 second

RHYTHM IDENTIFICATION

Sinus bradycardia with 6-second episode of sinus arrest and a PVC
- ◆ Ventricular rhythm   Irregular
- ◆ Ventricular rate   0 to 47/min (sinus beats)
- ◆ Atrial rhythm   Irregular
- ◆ Atrial rate   0 to 47/min (sinus beats)
- ◆ PRI: 0.18 second (sinus beats)
- ◆ QRS: 0.08 second (sinus beats)

RHYTHM IDENTIFICATION

Sinus tachycardia with PACs
- ◆ Ventricular rhythm   Regular except for the event
- ◆ Ventricular rate   136/min (sinus beats)
- ◆ Atrial rhythm   Regular except for the event
- ◆ Atrial rate   136/min (sinus beats)
- ◆ PRI: 0.12 to 0.14 second (sinus beats)
- ◆ QRS: 0.12 second (sinus beats)

RHYTHM IDENTIFICATION

- This rhythm strip is from an 82-year-old man with an altered level of responsiveness. Although a weak pulse is present, a blood pressure is not palpable. His skin is cool, pale, and moist. Identify the rhythm (lead II).

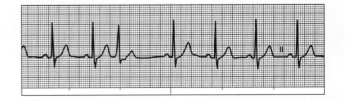

RHYTHM IDENTIFICATION

- Identify the rhythm.

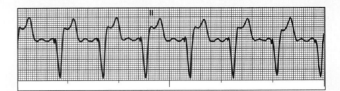

RHYTHM IDENTIFICATION

- This rhythm strip is from a 25-year-old man with a 4-week history of pneumonia. Identify the rhythm (lead II).

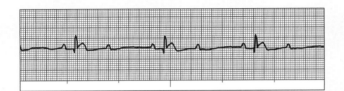

RHYTHM IDENTIFICATION

- This rhythm strip is from a 53-year-old woman with an altered level of responsiveness. Identify the rhythm (lead II).

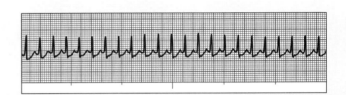

RHYTHM IDENTIFICATION

- These rhythm strips are from a 69-year-old woman found unresponsive, apneic, and pulseless. Identify the rhythm.

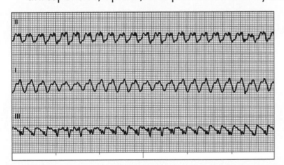

RHYTHM IDENTIFICATION

- This rhythm strip is from a 90-year-old woman with difficulty breathing. Identify the rhythm (lead II).

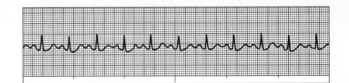

RHYTHM IDENTIFICATION

- Identify the rhythm (lead II).

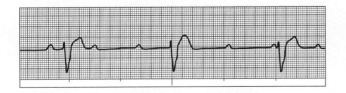

RHYTHM IDENTIFICATION

- Identify the rhythm.

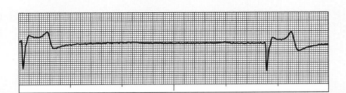

RHYTHM IDENTIFICATION

100% ventricular paced rhythm
- Atrial paced activity?   No
- Ventricular paced activity?   Yes
- Paced interval rate?   68

RHYTHM IDENTIFICATION

Agonal rhythm
- Ventricular rhythm   Regular
- Ventricular rate   13/min
- Atrial rhythm   Unable to determine
- Atrial rate   Unable to determine
- PRI: Unable to determine
- QRS: 0.12 second

RHYTHM IDENTIFICATION

Narrow-QRS tachycardia (supraventricular tachycardia [SVT]) with ST-segment depression
- Ventricular rhythm   Regular
- Ventricular rate   233/min
- Atrial rhythm   Unable to determine
- Atrial rate   Unable to determine
- PRI: Unable to determine
- QRS: 0.06 second

RHYTHM IDENTIFICATION

Second-degree AV block, 2:1 conduction, probably type I
- Ventricular rhythm   Regular
- Ventricular rate   35/min
- Atrial rhythm   Regular
- Atrial rate   70/min
- PRI: 0.24 to 0.26 second
- QRS: 0.08 to 0.10 second

RHYTHM IDENTIFICATION

Sinus tachycardia
- Ventricular rhythm   Regular
- Ventricular rate   111/min
- Atrial rhythm   Regular
- Atrial rate   111/min
- PRI: 0.16 second
- QRS: 0.04 to 0.06 second

RHYTHM IDENTIFICATION

Monomorphic ventricular tachycardia
- Ventricular rhythm   Regular
- Ventricular rate   225/min
- Atrial rhythm   Unable to determine
- Atrial rate   Unable to determine
- PRI: Unable to determine
- QRS: 0.14 second

RHYTHM IDENTIFICATION

Sinus rhythm with a PJC
- Ventricular rhythm   Regular except for the event
- Ventricular rate   75/min (sinus beats)
- Atrial rhythm   Regular except for the event
- Atrial rate   75/min (sinus beats)
- PRI: 0.16 second (sinus beats)
- QRS: 0.08 second

RHYTHM IDENTIFICATION

Complete (third-degree) AV block with ST-segment elevation
- Ventricular rhythm   Regular
- Ventricular rate   29/min
- Atrial rhythm   Regular
- Atrial rate   75/min
- PRI: Varies
- QRS: 0.14 second

RHYTHM IDENTIFICATION

◆ This rhythm strip is from a 14-year-old complaining of chest pain. Identify the rhythm.

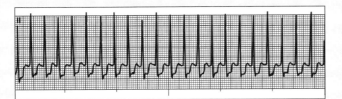

RHYTHM IDENTIFICATION

◆ This rhythm strip is from a 78-year-old woman complaining of left upper quadrant abdominal pain. Blood pressure 222/92. Blood sugar is 323. Identify the rhythm.

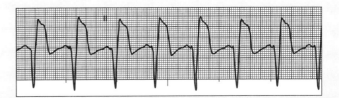

RHYTHM IDENTIFICATION

◆ This rhythm strip is from a 14-year-old complaining of chest pain. The following rhythm was observed on the monitor after 6 mg of adenosine IV. Identify the rhythm.

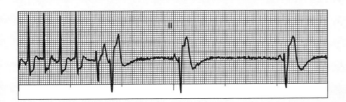

RHYTHM IDENTIFICATION

◆ Identify the rhythm (lead II).

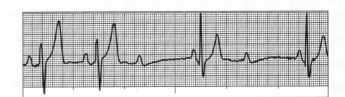

RHYTHM IDENTIFICATION

◆ This rhythm strip is from a 61-year-old man who experienced a syncopal episode. Blood pressure 105/86. Blood sugar is 131. Identify the rhythm.

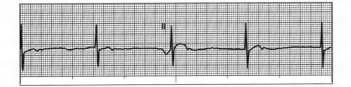

RHYTHM IDENTIFICATION

◆ This rhythm strip is from a 68-year-old woman complaining of chest pain and palpitations. She has a history of a prior myocardial infarction and COPD. Identify the rhythm (lead II).

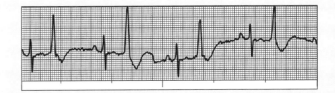

RHYTHM IDENTIFICATION

◆ This rhythm strip is from an 86-year-old woman complaining of dizziness. Identify the rhythm (lead II).

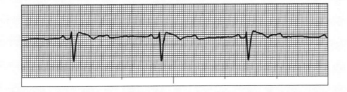

RHYTHM IDENTIFICATION

◆ This rhythm strip is from a 50-year-old man that awoke with shortness of breath. Lung sounds are clear bilaterally. Blood pressure 142/78. Identify the rhythm (lead II).

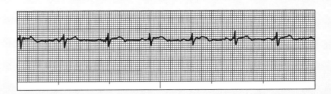

RHYTHM IDENTIFICATION

Sinus rhythm with ST-segment elevation
- Ventricular rhythm   Regular
- Ventricular rate   86/min
- Atrial rhythm   Regular
- Atrial rate   86/min
- PRI: 0.18 to 0.20 second
- QRS: 0.10 second

RHYTHM IDENTIFICATION

Narrow-QRS tachycardia (supraventricular tachycardia [SVT]) with ST-segment depression
- Ventricular rhythm   Regular
- Ventricular rate   214/min
- Atrial rhythm   Unable to determine
- Atrial rate   Unable to determine
- PRI: Unable to determine
- QRS: 0.06 second

RHYTHM IDENTIFICATION

Sinus bradycardia to second-degree AV block type II
- Ventricular rhythm   Irregular
- Ventricular rate   30/min
- Atrial rhythm   Regular
- Atrial rate   59/min
- PRI: 0.16 second
- QRS: 0.12 second

RHYTHM IDENTIFICATION

Narrow-QRS tachycardia (SVT) with ST-segment depression—sinus beat—PVC—sinus bradycardia
- Ventricular rhythm   Regular (SVT) to irregular as rhythm conversion occurs
- Ventricular rate   214/min (SVT) to 28 to 39 (sinus beats)
- Atrial rhythm   Unable to determine (SVT) to irregular (sinus beats)
- Atrial rate   Unable to determine (SVT) to 28 to 39 (sinus beats)
- PRI: Unable to determine (SVT) to 0.12 to 0.16 (sinus beats)
- QRS: 0.06 second (SVT) 0.06 (in last sinus beat)

RHYTHM IDENTIFICATION

Sinus bradycardia with ventricular bigeminy
- Ventricular rhythm   Regular except for the event (every other beat is an ectopic beat)
- Ventricular rate   42/min (sinus beats)
- Atrial rhythm   Regular except for the event
- Atrial rate   42/min (sinus beats)
- PRI: 0.16 to 0.20 second (sinus beats)
- QRS: 0.12 second (sinus beats)

RHYTHM IDENTIFICATION

Junctional escape rhythm
- Ventricular rhythm   Regular
- Ventricular rate   42/min
- Atrial rhythm   None
- Atrial rate   None
- PRI: None
- QRS: 0.06 to 0.08 second

RHYTHM IDENTIFICATION

Sinus rhythm
- Ventricular rhythm   Regular
- Ventricular rate   73/min
- Atrial rhythm   Regular
- Atrial rate   73/min
- PRI: 0.18 to 0.20 second
- QRS: 0.10 second

RHYTHM IDENTIFICATION

Second-degree AV block, 2:1 conduction, probably type II
- Ventricular rhythm   Regular
- Ventricular rate   35/min
- Atrial rhythm   Regular
- Atrial rate   70/min
- PRI: 0.20 second
- QRS: 0.12 second

RHYTHM IDENTIFICATION

◆ This rhythm strip is from a 26-year-old man after a seizure. Identify the rhythm (lead II).

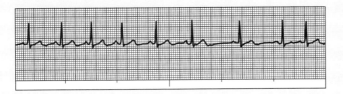

RHYTHM IDENTIFICATION

◆ This rhythm strip is from an 80-year-old woman complaining of chest pain after a motor vehicle crash. Blood pressure 140/90. Identify the rhythm (lead II).

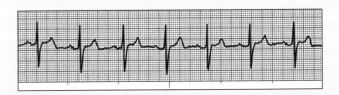

RHYTHM IDENTIFICATION

◆ This rhythm strip is from an 84-year-old man who was injured in a ground level fall. Identify the rhythm (lead II).

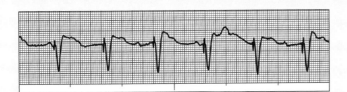

RHYTHM IDENTIFICATION

◆ This rhythm strip is from a 78-year-old woman complaining of chest pain. Identify the rhythm (lead II).

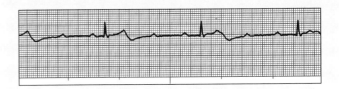

RHYTHM IDENTIFICATION

◆ Identify the rhythm (lead II).

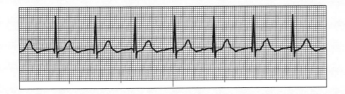

RHYTHM IDENTIFICATION

◆ This rhythm strip is from a 45-year-old man complaining of chest pain that he rates a 9 on a 1 to 10 scale. Blood pressure 88/P. Identify the rhythm (lead II).

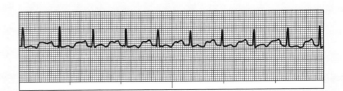

RHYTHM IDENTIFICATION

◆ Identify the rhythm (lead I).

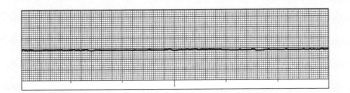

RHYTHM IDENTIFICATION

◆ Identify the rhythm (lead II).

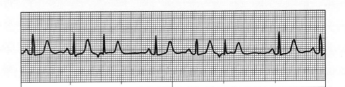

RHYTHM IDENTIFICATION

Sinus rhythm
- Ventricular rhythm   Regular
- Ventricular rate   71/min
- Atrial rhythm   Regular
- Atrial rate   71/min
- PRI: 0.20 second
- QRS: 0.10 second

RHYTHM IDENTIFICATION

Sinus arrhythmia
- Ventricular rhythm   Irregular
- Ventricular rate   64 to 94/min
- Atrial rhythm   Irregular
- Atrial rate   64 to 94/min
- PRI: 0.16 second
- QRS: 0.06 to 0.08 second

RHYTHM IDENTIFICATION

Complete (third-degree) AV block
- Ventricular rhythm   Regular
- Ventricular rate   32/min
- Atrial rhythm   Regular
- Atrial rate   100/min
- PRI: Varies
- QRS: 0.06 to 0.08 second

RHYTHM IDENTIFICATION

100% ventricular paced rhythm
- Atrial paced activity?   No
- Ventricular paced activity?   Yes
- Paced interval rate?   64

RHYTHM IDENTIFICATION

Sinus rhythm with inverted T waves
- Ventricular rhythm   Regular
- Ventricular rate   94/min
- Atrial rhythm   Regular
- Atrial rate   94/min
- PRI: 0.20 second
- QRS: 0.06 second

RHYTHM IDENTIFICATION

Accelerated junctional rhythm
- Ventricular rhythm   Regular
- Ventricular rate   79/min
- Atrial rhythm   None
- Atrial rate   None
- PRI: None
- QRS: 0.06 second

RHYTHM IDENTIFICATION

Sinus rhythm with PJCs
- Ventricular rhythm   Regular except for the event(s)
- Ventricular rate   77/min (sinus beats)
- Atrial rhythm   Regular except for the event(s)
- Atrial rate   77/min (sinus beats)
- PRI: 0.16 second (sinus beats)
- QRS: 0.04 to 0.06 second (sinus beats)

RHYTHM IDENTIFICATION

P-wave asystole
- Ventricular rhythm   None
- Ventricular rate   None
- Atrial rhythm   Regular
- Atrial rate   38/min
- PRI: None
- QRS: None

RHYTHM IDENTIFICATION

◆ Identify the rhythm (lead II).

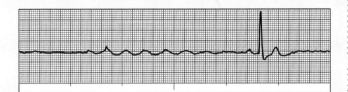

RHYTHM IDENTIFICATION

◆ This rhythm strip is from an 83-year-old man with rectal bleeding. Identify the rhythm (lead II).

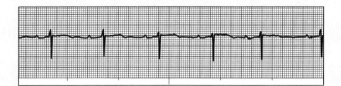

RHYTHM IDENTIFICATION

◆ This rhythm strip is from a 72-year-old man complaining of nausea and lightheadedness. He suffered a stroke 2 months ago. Identify the rhythm (lead II).

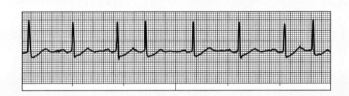

RHYTHM IDENTIFICATION

◆ This rhythm strip is from a 58-year-old woman complaining of palpitations. Blood pressure 130/91. Identify the rhythm (lead II).

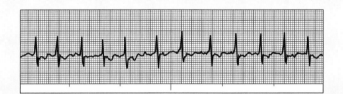

RHYTHM IDENTIFICATION

◆ Identify the rhythm (lead II).

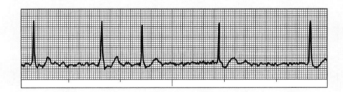

RHYTHM IDENTIFICATION

◆ These rhythm strips are from a 41-year-old woman complaining of difficulty breathing and a headache. She has a history of hypertension and had a coronary artery bypass graft 6 months ago. Identify the rhythm.

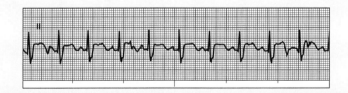

RHYTHM IDENTIFICATION

◆ This rhythm strip is from a 62-year-old unresponsive patient with diabetes. Identify the rhythm (lead II).

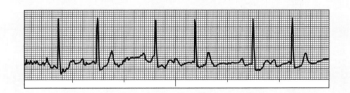

RHYTHM IDENTIFICATION

◆ Identify the rhythm (lead II).

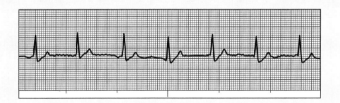

RHYTHM IDENTIFICATION

Sinus bradycardia with first-degree AV block
- ◆ Ventricular rhythm — Regular
- ◆ Ventricular rate — 57/min
- ◆ Atrial rhythm — Regular
- ◆ Atrial rate — 57/min
- ◆ PRI: — 0.28 second
- ◆ QRS: — 0.08 second

RHYTHM IDENTIFICATION

Ventricular fibrillation to sinus beat, ST-segment depression
- ◆ Ventricular rhythm — None to a single sinus beat
- ◆ Ventricular rate — Unable to determine
- ◆ Atrial rhythm — None to a single sinus beat
- ◆ Atrial rate — Unable to determine
- ◆ PRI: — 0.24 second (sinus beat)
- ◆ QRS: — 0.08 second (sinus beat)

RHYTHM IDENTIFICATION

Atrial fibrillation (uncontrolled)
- ◆ Ventricular rhythm — Irregular
- ◆ Ventricular rate — 100 to 150/min
- ◆ Atrial rhythm — Unable to determine
- ◆ Atrial rate — Unable to determine
- ◆ PRI: — Unable to determine
- ◆ QRS: — 0.08 to 0.10 second

RHYTHM IDENTIFICATION

Sinus rhythm with two PACs, ST-segment depression
- ◆ Ventricular rhythm — Regular except for the events
- ◆ Ventricular rate — 68/min (sinus beats)
- ◆ Atrial rhythm — Regular except for the events
- ◆ Atrial rate — 68/min (sinus beats)
- ◆ PRI: — 0.20 second (sinus beats)
- ◆ QRS: — 0.06 second (sinus beats)

RHYTHM IDENTIFICATION

Sinus tachycardia with ST-segment elevation
- ◆ Ventricular rhythm — Regular
- ◆ Ventricular rate — 107/min
- ◆ Atrial rhythm — Regular
- ◆ Atrial rate — 107/min
- ◆ PRI: — 0.16 second
- ◆ QRS: — 0.08 to 0.12 second

RHYTHM IDENTIFICATION

Atrial fibrillation (controlled)
- ◆ Ventricular rhythm — Irregular
- ◆ Ventricular rate — 34 to 75/min
- ◆ Atrial rhythm — Unable to determine
- ◆ Atrial rate — Unable to determine
- ◆ PRI: — Unable to determine
- ◆ QRS: — 0.08 second

RHYTHM IDENTIFICATION

Accelerated junctional rhythm with ST-segment depression
- ◆ Ventricular rhythm — Regular
- ◆ Ventricular rate — 69/min
- ◆ Atrial rhythm — Regular
- ◆ Atrial rate — 69/min
- ◆ PRI: — 0.12 second
- ◆ QRS: — 0.08 to 0.10 second

RHYTHM IDENTIFICATION

Second-degree AV block type I with ST-segment depression
- ◆ Ventricular rhythm — Irregular
- ◆ Ventricular rate — 54 to 79/min
- ◆ Atrial rhythm — Regular
- ◆ Atrial rate — 100/min
- ◆ PRI: — Lengthens
- ◆ QRS: — 0.06 second

RHYTHM IDENTIFICATION

◆ Identify the rhythm (lead II).

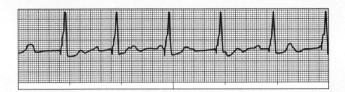

RHYTHM IDENTIFICATION

◆ This rhythm strip is from an 82-year-old woman that suffered a ground level fall. Blood pressure 110/72. Blood sugar is 156. Identify the rhythm (lead II).

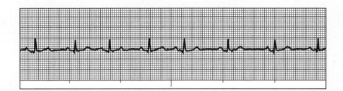

RHYTHM IDENTIFICATION

◆ Identify the rhythm (lead II).

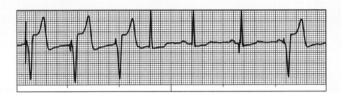

RHYTHM IDENTIFICATION

◆ This rhythm strip is from a 75-year-old man complaining of difficulty breathing. Blood pressure 190/130. Identify the rhythm (lead II).

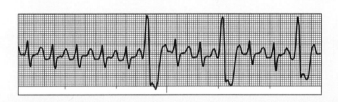

RHYTHM IDENTIFICATION

◆ Identify the rhythm (lead II).

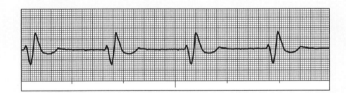

RHYTHM IDENTIFICATION

◆ This rhythm strip is from a 57-year-old man who collapsed on the golf course. He is unresponsive, apneic, and pulseless. Identify the rhythm.

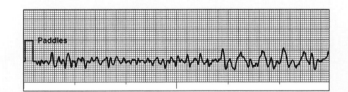

RHYTHM IDENTIFICATION

◆ Identify the rhythm (lead II).

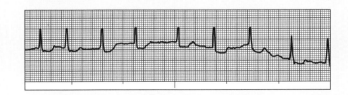

RHYTHM IDENTIFICATION

◆ This rhythm strip is from a 25-year-old man with an altered level of responsiveness due to ingestion of alcohol. Identify the rhythm (lead II).

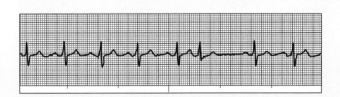

Sinus rhythm with PACs
- Ventricular rhythm — Regular except for the event
- Ventricular rate — 79/min (sinus beats)
- Atrial rhythm — Regular except for the event
- Atrial rate — 79/min (sinus beats)
- PRI: — 0.16 second
- QRS: — 0.06 second

Complete (third-degree) AV block with ST-segment depression
- Ventricular rhythm — Regular
- Ventricular rate — 60/min
- Atrial rhythm — Regular
- Atrial rate — 115/min
- PRI: — Varies
- QRS: — 0.14 second

Sinus tachycardia with a first-degree AV block, wide QRS, and uniform PVCs
- Ventricular rhythm — Regular except for the event
- Ventricular rate — 125/min (sinus beats)
- Atrial rhythm — Regular except for the event
- Atrial rate — 125/min (sinus beats)
- PRI: — 0.22 second (sinus beats)
- QRS: — 0.12 to 0.14 second (sinus beats)

Sinus rhythm with a ventricular demand pacer
- Atrial paced activity? — No
- Ventricular paced activity? — Yes
- Paced interval rate? — 68

Ventricular fibrillation
- Ventricular rhythm — None
- Ventricular rate — None
- Atrial rhythm — None
- Atrial rate — None
- PRI: — None
- QRS: — None

Idioventricular (ventricular escape) rhythm
- Ventricular rhythm — Regular
- Ventricular rate — 38/min
- Atrial rhythm — None
- Atrial rate — None
- PRI: — None
- QRS: — 0.18 second

Sinus rhythm with a PAC
- Ventricular rhythm — Regular except for the event
- Ventricular rate — 81/min
- Atrial rhythm — Regular except for the event
- Atrial rate — 81/min
- PRI: — 0.18 second
- QRS: — 0.10 second

Atrial fibrillation
- Ventricular rhythm — Irregular
- Ventricular rate — 71 to 115/min
- Atrial rhythm — Unable to determine
- Atrial rate — Unable to determine
- PRI: — Unable to determine
- QRS: — 0.06 to 0.08 second

RHYTHM IDENTIFICATION

◆ This rhythm strip is from a 34-year-old woman complaining of palpitations. She has no significant past medical history. Identify the rhythm (lead II).

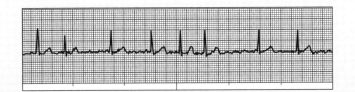

RHYTHM IDENTIFICATION

◆ Identify the rhythm (lead II).

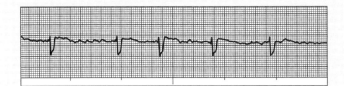

RHYTHM IDENTIFICATION

◆ Identify the rhythm.

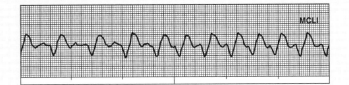

RHYTHM IDENTIFICATION

◆ Identify the rhythm (lead II).

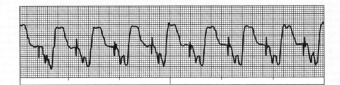

RHYTHM IDENTIFICATION

◆ Identify the rhythm (lead II).

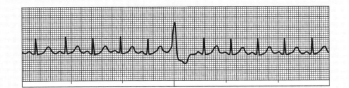

RHYTHM IDENTIFICATION

◆ Identify the rhythm (lead II).

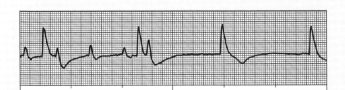

RHYTHM IDENTIFICATION

◆ This rhythm strip is from a 35-year-old woman who attempted suicide. Blood pressure 118/80, respirations 16. Identify the rhythm (lead II).

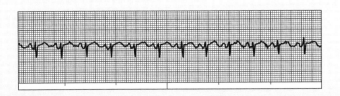

RHYTHM IDENTIFICATION

◆ Identify the rhythm (top = lead II, middle = lead I, bottom = lead III).

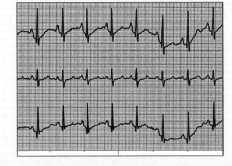

RHYTHM IDENTIFICATION

Atrial fibrillation (controlled) with a wide-QRS
- Ventricular rhythm   Irregular
- Ventricular rate   47 to 73/min
- Atrial rhythm   Unable to determine
- Atrial rate   Unable to determine
- PRI: Unable to determine
- QRS: 0.12 second

RHYTHM IDENTIFICATION

Atrial fibrillation
- Ventricular rhythm   Irregular
- Ventricular rate   57 to 125/min
- Atrial rhythm   Unable to determine
- Atrial rate   Unable to determine
- PRI: Unable to determine
- QRS: 0.08 second

RHYTHM IDENTIFICATION

100% ventricular paced rhythm
- Atrial paced activity?   No
- Ventricular paced activity?   Yes
- Paced interval rate?   80

RHYTHM IDENTIFICATION

Wide-complex tachycardia of uncertain origin
- Ventricular rhythm   Irregular
- Ventricular rate   115/min
- Atrial rhythm   Unable to determine
- Atrial rate   Unable to determine
- PRI: Unable to determine
- QRS: 0.14 to 0.16 second

RHYTHM IDENTIFICATION

Complete (third-degree) AV block to an idioventricular (ventricular escape) rhythm
- Ventricular rhythm   Regular
- Ventricular rate   32/min
- Atrial rhythm   Regular
- Atrial rate   91/min
- PRI: Varies
- QRS: 0.16 to 0.18 second

RHYTHM IDENTIFICATION

Sinus tachycardia with a PVC
- Ventricular rhythm   Regular except for the event
- Ventricular rate   111/min (sinus beats)
- Atrial rhythm   Regular except for the event
- Atrial rate   111/min (sinus beats)
- PRI: 0.16 second
- QRS: 0.04 second

RHYTHM IDENTIFICATION

Sinus rhythm
- Ventricular rhythm   Regular
- Ventricular rate   79/min
- Atrial rhythm   Regular
- Atrial rate   79/min
- PRI: 0.16 second
- QRS: 0.06 second

RHYTHM IDENTIFICATION

Sinus tachycardia with ST-segment elevation
- Ventricular rhythm   Regular
- Ventricular rate   130/min
- Atrial rhythm   Regular
- Atrial rate   130/min
- PRI: 0.16 second
- QRS: 0.08 second

RHYTHM IDENTIFICATION

◆ This rhythm strip is from a 63-year-old woman complaining of dizziness. Identify the rhythm (lead II).

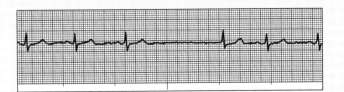

RHYTHM IDENTIFICATION

◆ Identify the rhythm (lead II).

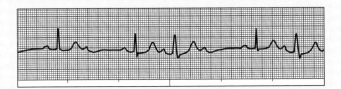

RHYTHM IDENTIFICATION

◆ Identify the rhythm.

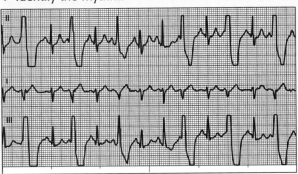

RHYTHM IDENTIFICATION

◆ This rhythm strip is from a 62-year-old man complaining of palpitations. Identify the rhythm (lead II).

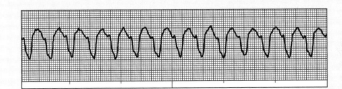

RHYTHM IDENTIFICATION

◆ Identify the rhythm (lead II).

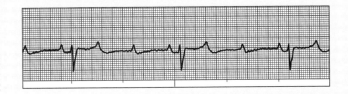

RHYTHM IDENTIFICATION

◆ This rhythm strip is from a 62-year-old man complaining of palpitations. A synchronized shock was delivered, resulting in the following rhythm. Identify the rhythm (lead II).

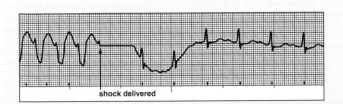

shock delivered

RHYTHM IDENTIFICATION

◆ Identify the rhythm.

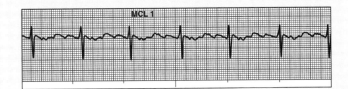

MCL 1

RHYTHM IDENTIFICATION

◆ These rhythm strips are from a 44-year-old woman complaining of chest pain. Identify the rhythm.

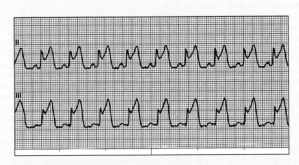

RHYTHM IDENTIFICATION

RHYTHM IDENTIFICATION

Second-degree AV block type I
- Ventricular rhythm — Irregular
- Ventricular rate — 37 to 79/min
- Atrial rhythm — Regular
- Atrial rate — 79/min
- PRI: — Lengthens
- QRS: — 0.06 to 0.10 second

Sinus rhythm with a 2.6-second episode of sinus arrest and a junctional escape beat
- Ventricular rhythm — Regular except for the event
- Ventricular rate — 64/min (sinus beats)
- Atrial rhythm — Regular except for the event
- Atrial rate — 64/min (sinus beats)
- PRI: — 0.16 to 0.18 second
- QRS: — 0.08 second

RHYTHM IDENTIFICATION

RHYTHM IDENTIFICATION

Monomorphic ventricular tachycardia
- Ventricular rhythm — Regular
- Ventricular rate — 150/min
- Atrial rhythm — Unable to determine
- Atrial rate — Unable to determine
- PRI: — Unable to determine
- QRS: — 0.16 second

Sinus tachycardia with frequent uniform PVCs
- Ventricular rhythm — Regular
- Ventricular rate — 150/min (sinus beats)
- Atrial rhythm — Regular
- Atrial rate — 150/min (sinus beats)
- PRI: — 0.16 second (sinus beats)
- QRS: — 0.08 second (sinus beats)

RHYTHM IDENTIFICATION

RHYTHM IDENTIFICATION

Monomorphic ventricular tachycardia to sinus rhythm with first-degree AV block
- Ventricular rhythm — Regular (sinus beats)
- Ventricular rate — 97/min (sinus beats)
- Atrial rhythm — Regular (sinus beats)
- Atrial rate — 97/min (sinus beats)
- PRI: — 0.22 second (sinus beats)
- QRS: — 0.10 second (sinus beats)

Second-degree AV block type II
- Ventricular rhythm — Regular
- Ventricular rate — 29/min
- Atrial rhythm — Regular
- Atrial rate — 88/min
- PRI: — 0.22 second
- QRS: — 0.12 second

RHYTHM IDENTIFICATION

RHYTHM IDENTIFICATION

Sinus rhythm with ST-segment elevation
- Ventricular rhythm — Regular
- Ventricular rate — 94/min
- Atrial rhythm — Regular
- Atrial rate — 94/min
- PRI: — 0.16 second
- QRS: — 0.08 second

Atrial flutter
- Ventricular rhythm — Regular
- Ventricular rate — 65/min
- Atrial rhythm — Unable to determine
- Atrial rate — Unable to determine
- PRI: — Unable to determine
- QRS: — 0.10 second

RHYTHM IDENTIFICATION

◆ Identify the rhythm (lead II).

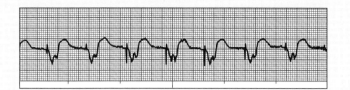

RHYTHM IDENTIFICATION

◆ Identify the rhythm.

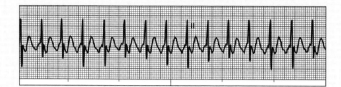

RHYTHM IDENTIFICATION

◆ Identify the rhythm (lead II).

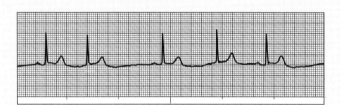

RHYTHM IDENTIFICATION

◆ Identify the rhythm.

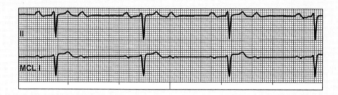

RHYTHM IDENTIFICATION

◆ Identify the rhythm (lead II).

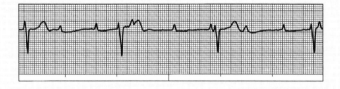

RHYTHM IDENTIFICATION

◆ Identify the rhythm (lead II).

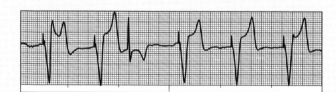

RHYTHM IDENTIFICATION

◆ Identify the rhythm (lead II).

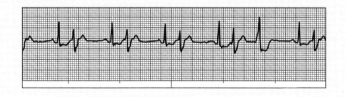

RHYTHM IDENTIFICATION

◆ Identify the rhythm (lead II).

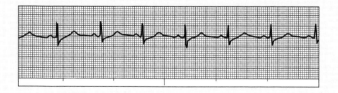

RHYTHM IDENTIFICATION

Atrial flutter (2:1 conduction)
- Ventricular rhythm   Regular
- Ventricular rate   150/min
- Atrial rhythm   Unable to determine
- Atrial rate   Unable to determine
- PRI: Unable to determine
- QRS: 0.08 second

RHYTHM IDENTIFICATION

100% ventricular paced rhythm
- Atrial paced activity?   No
- Ventricular paced activity?   Yes
- Paced interval rate?   80

RHYTHM IDENTIFICATION

Second-degree AV block, 2:1 conduction, probably type I
- Ventricular rhythm   Regular
- Ventricular rate   36/min
- Atrial rhythm   Regular
- Atrial rate   75/min
- PRI: 0.32 second
- QRS: 0.10 second

RHYTHM IDENTIFICATION

Sinus bradycardia with a PJC
- Ventricular rhythm   Regular except for the event
- Ventricular rate   52/min (sinus beats)
- Atrial rhythm   Regular except for the event
- Atrial rate   52/min (sinus beats)
- PRI: 0.16 second (sinus beats)
- QRS: 0.06 second

RHYTHM IDENTIFICATION

Ventricular demand pacer
- Atrial paced activity?   No
- Ventricular paced activity?   Yes
- Paced interval rate?   60

RHYTHM IDENTIFICATION

Complete (third-degree) AV block
- Ventricular rhythm   Regular
- Ventricular rate   32/min
- Atrial rhythm   Regular
- Atrial rate   83/min
- PRI: Varies
- QRS: 0.12 second

RHYTHM IDENTIFICATION

Sinus rhythm
- Ventricular rhythm   Regular
- Ventricular rate   75/min
- Atrial rhythm   Regular
- Atrial rate   75/min
- PRI: 0.16 second
- QRS: 0.08 second

RHYTHM IDENTIFICATION

Sinus bradycardia with ventricular bigeminy
- Ventricular rhythm   Regular except for the event (every other beat is an ectopic beat)
- Ventricular rate   58/min (sinus beats)
- Atrial rhythm   Regular except for the event
- Atrial rate   58/min (sinus beats)
- PRI: 0.16 second (sinus beats)
- QRS: 0.06 second (sinus beats)

RHYTHM IDENTIFICATION

◆ This rhythm strip is from a 29-year-old woman with a kidney stone. Identify the rhythm (lead II).

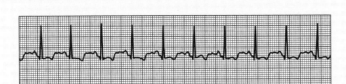

RHYTHM IDENTIFICATION

◆ Identify the rhythm.

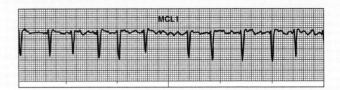

RHYTHM IDENTIFICATION

◆ Identify the rhythm (lead II).

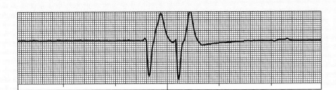

RHYTHM IDENTIFICATION

◆ This rhythm strip is from a 78-year-old man found unresponsive, apneic, and pulseless. Identify the rhythm (lead II).

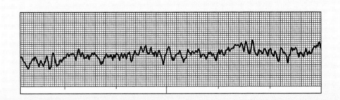

RHYTHM IDENTIFICATION

◆ Identify the rhythm (lead II).

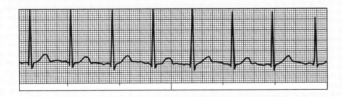

RHYTHM IDENTIFICATION

◆ This rhythm strip is from an 82-year-old woman with an altered level of responsiveness. Identify the rhythm (lead II).

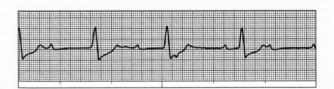

RHYTHM IDENTIFICATION

◆ Identify the rhythm (lead II).

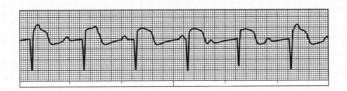

RHYTHM IDENTIFICATION

◆ This rhythm strip is from a 59-year-old man who was driving to work on the freeway when his internal defibrillator discharged. He was asymptomatic at the time this ECG was obtained a few minutes after the event. Identify the rhythm (lead II).

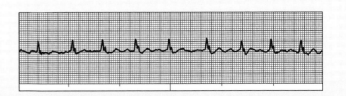

Atrial fibrillation
- ◆ Ventricular rhythm   Irregular
- ◆ Ventricular rate   71 to 150/min
- ◆ Atrial rhythm   Unable to determine
- ◆ Atrial rate   Unable to determine
- ◆ PRI: Unable to determine
- ◆ QRS: 0.08 to 0.10 second

Sinus tachycardia with inverted T waves
- ◆ Ventricular rhythm   Regular
- ◆ Ventricular rate   103/min
- ◆ Atrial rhythm   Regular
- ◆ Atrial rate   103/min
- ◆ PRI: 0.14 second
- ◆ QRS: 0.08 second

Ventricular fibrillation
- ◆ Ventricular rhythm   None
- ◆ Ventricular rate   None
- ◆ Atrial rhythm   None
- ◆ Atrial rate   None
- ◆ PRI: None
- ◆ QRS: None

Agonal rhythm/asystole
- ◆ Ventricular rhythm   Two ventricular complexes to none
- ◆ Ventricular rate   None
- ◆ Atrial rhythm   None
- ◆ Atrial rate   None
- ◆ PRI: None
- ◆ QRS: 0.14 second to none

Complete (third-degree) AV block with ST-segment depression
- ◆ Ventricular rhythm   Regular
- ◆ Ventricular rate   39/min
- ◆ Atrial rhythm   Regular
- ◆ Atrial rate   71/min
- ◆ PRI: Varies
- ◆ QRS: 0.16 second

Accelerated junctional rhythm
- ◆ Ventricular rhythm   Regular
- ◆ Ventricular rate   77/min
- ◆ Atrial rhythm   Regular
- ◆ Atrial rate   77/min
- ◆ PRI: 0.12 to 0.14 second
- ◆ QRS: 0.08 second

Atrial fibrillation
- ◆ Ventricular rhythm   Irregular
- ◆ Ventricular rate   83 to 115/min
- ◆ Atrial rhythm   Unable to determine
- ◆ Atrial rate   Unable to determine
- ◆ PRI: Unable to determine
- ◆ QRS: 0.08 to 0.10 second

Complete (third-degree) AV block with ST-segment elevation
- ◆ Ventricular rhythm   Regular
- ◆ Ventricular rate   60/min
- ◆ Atrial rhythm   Regular
- ◆ Atrial rate   114/min
- ◆ PRI: Varies
- ◆ QRS: 0.08 second

RHYTHM IDENTIFICATION

◆ This rhythm strip is from a 15-year-old boy with a stab wound to his chest. The patient was unresponsive, apneic, and pulseless. Identify the rhythm (lead II).

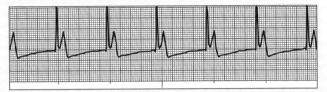

Time: 00:15:06

RHYTHM IDENTIFICATION

◆ This rhythm strip is from a 15-year-old boy with a stab wound to his chest. A pulse is present. Blood pressure is 90/P. Identify the rhythm (lead II).

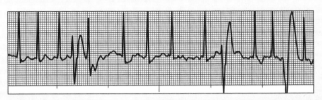

Time: 00:32:43

RHYTHM IDENTIFICATION

◆ This rhythm strip is from a 15-year-old boy with a stab wound to his chest. The patient was unresponsive, apneic, and pulseless. Identify the rhythm (lead II).

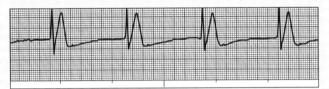

Time: 00:19:47

RHYTHM IDENTIFICATION

◆ Identify the rhythm.

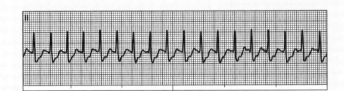

RHYTHM IDENTIFICATION

◆ This rhythm strip is from a 15-year-old boy with a stab wound to his chest. The patient was unresponsive, apneic, and pulseless. Identify the rhythm (lead II).

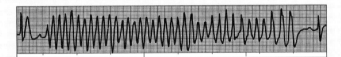

Time: 00:32:11

RHYTHM IDENTIFICATION

◆ Identify the rhythm.

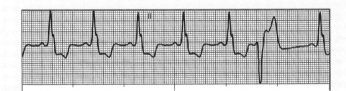

RHYTHM IDENTIFICATION

◆ This rhythm strip is from a 15-year-old boy with a stab wound to his chest. A pulse is present. Blood pressure is 90/P. Identify the rhythm (lead II).

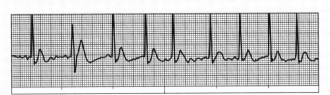

Time: 00:32:31

RHYTHM IDENTIFICATION

◆ Identify the rhythm (lead II).

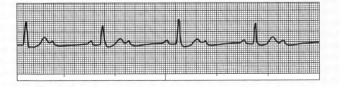

RHYTHM IDENTIFICATION

Atrial fibrillation with ventricular complexes
- ◆ Ventricular rhythm   Irregular
- ◆ Ventricular rate   71 to 167/min
- ◆ Atrial rhythm   Unable to determine
- ◆ Atrial rate   Unable to determine
- ◆ PRI: Unable to determine
- ◆ QRS: 0.06 second

RHYTHM IDENTIFICATION

Accelerated junctional rhythm with ST-segment elevation
- ◆ Ventricular rhythm   Regular
- ◆ Ventricular rate   62/min
- ◆ Atrial rhythm   Unable to determine
- ◆ Atrial rate   Unable to determine
- ◆ PRI: Unable to determine
- ◆ QRS: 0.06 second

RHYTHM IDENTIFICATION

Narrow-QRS tachycardia (supraventricular tachycardia [SVT]) with ST-segment depression
- ◆ Ventricular rhythm   Regular
- ◆ Ventricular rate   184/min
- ◆ Atrial rhythm   Unable to determine
- ◆ Atrial rate   Unable to determine
- ◆ PRI: Unable to determine
- ◆ QRS: 0.06 second

RHYTHM IDENTIFICATION

Junctional rhythm with tall T waves
- ◆ Ventricular rhythm   Regular
- ◆ Ventricular rate   40/min
- ◆ Atrial rhythm   Unable to determine
- ◆ Atrial rate   Unable to determine
- ◆ PRI: Unable to determine
- ◆ QRS: 0.06 second

RHYTHM IDENTIFICATION

Sinus rhythm with a wide-QRS and a PVC
- ◆ Ventricular rhythm   Regular except for the event
- ◆ Ventricular rate   68/min (sinus beats)
- ◆ Atrial rhythm   Regular except for the event
- ◆ Atrial rate   68/min (sinus beats)
- ◆ PRI: 0.16 second (sinus beats)
- ◆ QRS: 0.14 second (sinus beats)

RHYTHM IDENTIFICATION

Junctional beat to polymorphic VT to a sinus beat
- ◆ Ventricular rhythm   Irregular
- ◆ Ventricular rate   300/min (polymorphic VT)
- ◆ Atrial rhythm   Unable to determine
- ◆ Atrial rate   Unable to determine
- ◆ PRI: Unable to determine
- ◆ QRS: 0.14 (ventricular complexes) to 0.12 second (supraventricular complexes)

RHYTHM IDENTIFICATION

Second-degree AV block, 2:1 conduction, probably type I
- ◆ Ventricular rhythm   Regular
- ◆ Ventricular rate   41/min
- ◆ Atrial rhythm   Regular
- ◆ Atrial rate   79/min
- ◆ PRI: 0.24 second
- ◆ QRS: 0.08 to 0.10 second

RHYTHM IDENTIFICATION

Atrial fibrillation with a ventricular complex
- ◆ Ventricular rhythm   Irregular
- ◆ Ventricular rate   83 to 167/min
- ◆ Atrial rhythm   Unable to determine
- ◆ Atrial rate   Unable to determine
- ◆ PRI: Unable to determine
- ◆ QRS: 0.06 second

RHYTHM IDENTIFICATION

◆ This rhythm strip is from an 81-year-old woman with chest pain. Identify the rhythm.

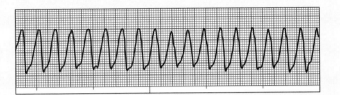

RHYTHM IDENTIFICATION

◆ Identify the rhythm (lead II).

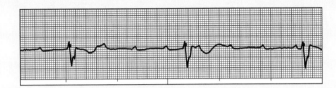

RHYTHM IDENTIFICATION

◆ Identify the rhythm (lead II).

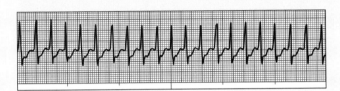

RHYTHM IDENTIFICATION

◆ This rhythm strip is from a 47-year-old man with an altered level of responsiveness. Blood pressure is 118/86. Blood sugar is 37. Identify the rhythm (lead II).

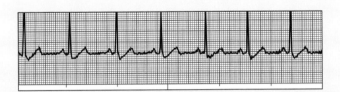

RHYTHM IDENTIFICATION

◆ Identify the rhythm (lead II).

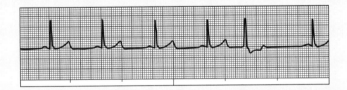

RHYTHM IDENTIFICATION

◆ Identify the rhythm.

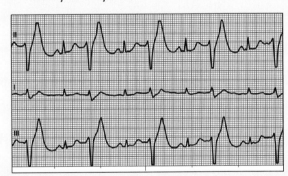

RHYTHM IDENTIFICATION

◆ Identify the rhythm (lead II).

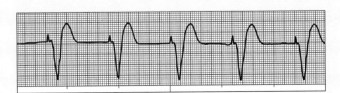

RHYTHM IDENTIFICATION

◆ This rhythm strip is from a 59-year-old woman found unresponsive, apneic, and pulseless. Identify the rhythm (lead III).

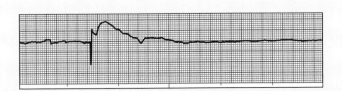

RHYTHM IDENTIFICATION

Complete (third-degree) AV block
- Ventricular rhythm — Regular
- Ventricular rate — 27/min
- Atrial rhythm — Regular
- Atrial rate — 107/min
- PRI: — Varies
- QRS: — 0.14 second

Treatment for a symptomatic patient with a complete AV block and a wide-QRS complex often includes use of a transcutaneous pacemaker until a transvenous or permanent pacemaker is inserted.

In this situation, the external pacemaker was applied. The pacemaker rate was set at 60, but no milliamps had been selected at the time the rhythm strip was recorded.

RHYTHM IDENTIFICATION

Monomorphic ventricular tachycardia
- Ventricular rhythm — Regular
- Ventricular rate — 214/min
- Atrial rhythm — Unable to determine
- Atrial rate — Unable to determine
- PRI: — Unable to determine
- QRS: — 0.16 to 0.18 second

RHYTHM IDENTIFICATION

Sinus rhythm with ST-segment depression
- Ventricular rhythm — Regular
- Ventricular rate — 68/min
- Atrial rhythm — Regular
- Atrial rate — 68/min
- PRI: — 0.16 second
- QRS: — 0.06 to 0.08 second

RHYTHM IDENTIFICATION

Narrow-QRS tachycardia (supraventricular tachycardia [SVT]) with ST-segment depression
- Ventricular rhythm — Regular
- Ventricular rate — 214/min
- Atrial rhythm — Unable to determine
- Atrial rate — Unable to determine
- PRI: — Unable to determine
- QRS: — 0.08 second

RHYTHM IDENTIFICATION

Sinus bradycardia with ventricular bigeminy
- Ventricular rhythm — Regular except for the event (every other beat is an ectopic beat)
- Ventricular rate — 44/min (sinus beats)
- Atrial rhythm — Regular except for the event
- Atrial rate — 44/min (sinus beats)
- PRI: — 0.20 second (sinus beats)
- QRS: — 0.06 second (sinus beats)

RHYTHM IDENTIFICATION

Sinus rhythm with a PJC
- Ventricular rhythm — Regular except for the event
- Ventricular rate — 60/min (sinus beats)
- Atrial rhythm — Regular except for the event
- Atrial rate — 60/min (sinus beats)
- PRI: — 0.14 second (sinus beats)
- QRS: — 0.06 second

RHYTHM IDENTIFICATION

Asystole
- Ventricular rhythm — None
- Ventricular rate — None
- Atrial rhythm — None
- Atrial rate — None
- PRI: — None
- QRS: — None

RHYTHM IDENTIFICATION

100% ventricular paced rhythm
- Atrial paced activity? — No
- Ventricular paced activity? — Yes
- Paced interval rate? — 52

RHYTHM IDENTIFICATION

◆ These rhythm strips are from a 24-year-old woman that attempted suicide. Blood pressure is 116/69. Identify the rhythm.

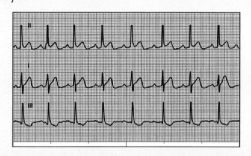

RHYTHM IDENTIFICATION

◆ This rhythm strip is a 71-year-old man complaining of abdominal pain. Identify the rhythm (lead II).

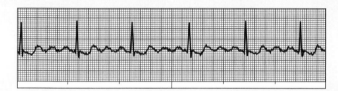

RHYTHM IDENTIFICATION

◆ This rhythm strip is from a 90-year-old unresponsive woman. She has a history of congestive heart failure. Her medications include furosemide and albuterol. Identify the rhythm (lead II).

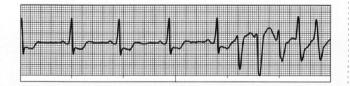

RHYTHM IDENTIFICATION

◆ This rhythm strip is from a 68-year-old woman who suffered a ground level fall. Identify the rhythm (lead II).

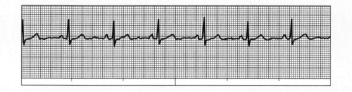

RHYTHM IDENTIFICATION

◆ This rhythm strip is from an 87-year-old woman complaining of "feeling ill." Identify the rhythm (lead II).

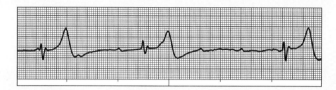

RHYTHM IDENTIFICATION

◆ These rhythm strips are from a 74-year-old man with difficulty breathing. Identify the rhythm (top = lead I, middle = lead II, bottom = lead III).

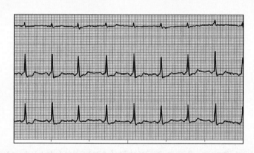

RHYTHM IDENTIFICATION

◆ Identify the rhythm (lead II).

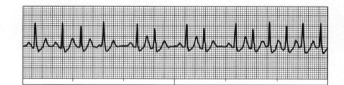

RHYTHM IDENTIFICATION

◆ This rhythm strip is from a 74-year-old man who is complaining of feeling lightheaded while sitting in church. His skin is cool and moist. Blood pressure is 118/68. He has a history of arthritis. Identify the rhythm (lead II).

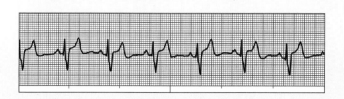

RHYTHM IDENTIFICATION

Complete (third-degree) AV block
- ◆ Ventricular rhythm   Regular
- ◆ Ventricular rate   30/min
- ◆ Atrial rhythm   Regular
- ◆ Atrial rate   80/min
- ◆ PRI: Varies
- ◆ QRS: 0.10 second

RHYTHM IDENTIFICATION

Sinus arrhythmia
- ◆ Ventricular rhythm   Irregular
- ◆ Ventricular rate   79 to 88/min
- ◆ Atrial rhythm   Irregular
- ◆ Atrial rate   79 to 88/min
- ◆ PRI: 0.18 second
- ◆ QRS: 0.08 second

RHYTHM IDENTIFICATION

Accelerated junctional rhythm with ST-segment depression
- ◆ Ventricular rhythm   Regular
- ◆ Ventricular rate   86/min
- ◆ Atrial rhythm   Regular
- ◆ Atrial rate   86/min
- ◆ PRI: 0.12 second
- ◆ QRS: 0.06 second

RHYTHM IDENTIFICATION

Atrial flutter
- ◆ Ventricular rhythm   Regular
- ◆ Ventricular rate   55/min
- ◆ Atrial rhythm   Unable to determine
- ◆ Atrial rate   Unable to determine
- ◆ PRI: Unable to determine
- ◆ QRS: 0.08 second

RHYTHM IDENTIFICATION

Sinus rhythm with PACs to narrow-QRS tachycardia
- ◆ Ventricular rhythm   Irregular to regular
- ◆ Ventricular rate   63/min (sinus beats) to 188/min
- ◆ Atrial rhythm   Irregular to unable to determine
- ◆ Atrial rate   63/min (sinus beats) to unable to determine
- ◆ PRI: 0.16 second (sinus beats) to unable to determine
- ◆ QRS: 0.06 second

RHYTHM IDENTIFICATION

Sinus rhythm with ST-segment depression to polymorphic ventricular tachycardia
- ◆ Ventricular rhythm   Regular (sinus beats) to irregular (ventricular beats)
- ◆ Ventricular rate   65/min (sinus beats) to approximately 167 (ventricular beats)
- ◆ Atrial rhythm   Regular (sinus beats)
- ◆ Atrial rate   65/min (sinus beats)
- ◆ PRI: 0.16 second (sinus beats)
- ◆ QRS: 0.10 to 0.12 second (sinus beats)

RHYTHM IDENTIFICATION

Sinus rhythm with a wide QRS and ST-segment elevation
- ◆ Ventricular rhythm   Regular
- ◆ Ventricular rate   68/min
- ◆ Atrial rhythm   Regular
- ◆ Atrial rate   68/min
- ◆ PRI: 0.16 second
- ◆ QRS: 0.12 second

RHYTHM IDENTIFICATION

Sinus rhythm
- ◆ Ventricular rhythm   Regular
- ◆ Ventricular rate   71/min
- ◆ Atrial rhythm   Regular
- ◆ Atrial rate   71/min
- ◆ PRI: 0.16 second
- ◆ QRS: 0.06 to 0.08 second

RHYTHM IDENTIFICATION

◆ This rhythm strip is from an 89-year-old man complaining of chest pain. He had a myocardial infarction 15 years ago and a coronary artery bypass graft 5 years ago. Blood pressure is 140/90. Identify the rhythm (lead II).

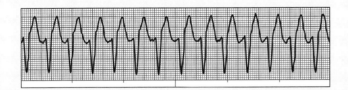

RHYTHM IDENTIFICATION

◆ Identify the rhythm (lead II).

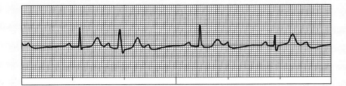

RHYTHM IDENTIFICATION

◆ Identify the rhythm (lead II).

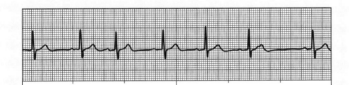

RHYTHM IDENTIFICATION

◆ Identify the rhythm (lead II).

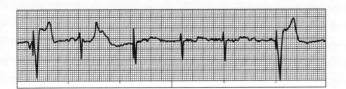

RHYTHM IDENTIFICATION

◆ Identify the rhythm (lead II).

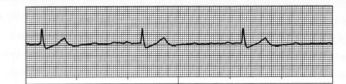

RHYTHM IDENTIFICATION

◆ This rhythm strip is from a 58-year-old man that was initially unresponsive, apneic, and pulseless. Identify the rhythm.

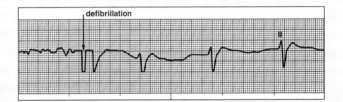

RHYTHM IDENTIFICATION

◆ This rhythm strip is from a 68-year-old man who suffered a head injury after a fall. Identify the rhythm (top = lead II, bottom = MCL1).

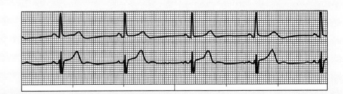

RHYTHM IDENTIFICATION

◆ Identify the rhythm (lead II).

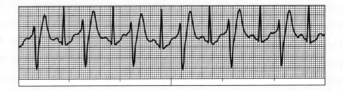

RHYTHM IDENTIFICATION

Second-degree AV block type II
- Ventricular rhythm — Regular
- Ventricular rate — 31/min
- Atrial rhythm — Regular
- Atrial rate — 31/min
- PRI: — 0.30 second
- QRS: — 0.08 to 0.10 second

RHYTHM IDENTIFICATION

Wide-complex tachycardia of uncertain origin
- Ventricular rhythm — Regular
- Ventricular rate — 136/min
- Atrial rhythm — Unable to determine
- Atrial rate — Unable to determine
- PRI: — Unable to determine
- QRS: — 0.10 to 0.14 second

RHYTHM IDENTIFICATION

Ventricular fibrillation—shock (defibrillation)—idioventricular (ventricular escape) rhythm
- Ventricular rhythm — Irregular to regular
- Ventricular rate — None to 40/min
- Atrial rhythm — None
- Atrial rate — None
- PRI: — None
- QRS: — None to 0.16 second

RHYTHM IDENTIFICATION

Second-degree AV block type I to 2:1 conduction
- Ventricular rhythm — Irregular
- Ventricular rate — 39 to 79/min
- Atrial rhythm — Regular
- Atrial rate — 79/min
- PRI: — Lengthens (2nd-degree type 1) to 0.24 second
- QRS: — 0.08 to 0.10 second

RHYTHM IDENTIFICATION

Sinus bradycardia
- Ventricular rhythm — Regular
- Ventricular rate — 51/min
- Atrial rhythm — Regular
- Atrial rate — 51/min
- PRI: — 0.16 second
- QRS: — 0.10 second

RHYTHM IDENTIFICATION

Sinus rhythm with a PAC and a nonconducted PAC
- Ventricular rhythm — Irregular
- Ventricular rate — 67 to 73/min (sinus beats)
- Atrial rhythm — Irregular
- Atrial rate — 67 to 73/min (sinus beats)
- PRI: — 0.16 second (sinus beats)
- QRS: — 0.08 second (sinus beats)

RHYTHM IDENTIFICATION

Sinus rhythm with ventricular bigeminy
- Ventricular rhythm — Regular except for the event (every other beat is an ectopic beat)
- Ventricular rate — 64/min (sinus beats)
- Atrial rhythm — Regular except for the event
- Atrial rate — 64/min (sinus beats)
- PRI: — 0.16 second (sinus beats)
- QRS: — 0.10 second (sinus beats)

RHYTHM IDENTIFICATION

Atrial fibrillation with a ventricular demand pacer
- Atrial paced activity? — No
- Ventricular paced activity? — Yes
- Paced interval rate? — 60

RHYTHM IDENTIFICATION

◆ Identify the rhythm.

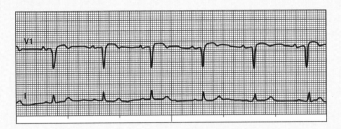

RHYTHM IDENTIFICATION

◆ Identify the rhythm (lead II).

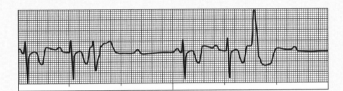

RHYTHM IDENTIFICATION

◆ Identify the rhythm (lead II).

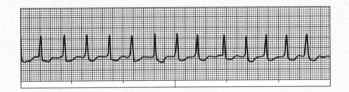

RHYTHM IDENTIFICATION

◆ This rhythm strip is from an asymptomatic 72-year-old man. Identify the rhythm.

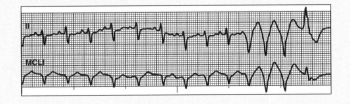

RHYTHM IDENTIFICATION

◆ This rhythm strip is from a 19-year-old man after a seizure. Identify the rhythm (lead II).

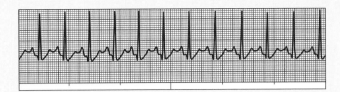

RHYTHM IDENTIFICATION

◆ This rhythm strip is from a 14-year-old complaining of chest pain. Identify the rhythm (lead II).

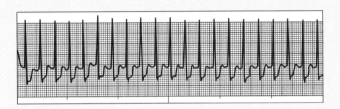

RHYTHM IDENTIFICATION

◆ This rhythm strip is from a 62-year-old man complaining of a sudden onset of sweating, nausea, and weakness. Blood pressure is 112/54. Blood sugar is 122. Identify the rhythm (lead II).

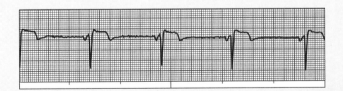

RHYTHM IDENTIFICATION

◆ This rhythm strip is from a 27-year-old asymptomatic woman. Identify the rhythm (lead II).

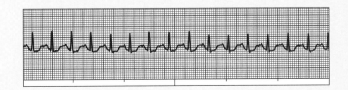

RHYTHM IDENTIFICATION

Sinus tachycardia
- Ventricular rhythm   Regular
- Ventricular rate   120/min
- Atrial rhythm   Regular
- Atrial rate   120/min
- PRI: 0.16 second
- QRS: 0.08 to 0.10 second

RHYTHM IDENTIFICATION

Sinus rhythm
- Ventricular rhythm   Regular
- Ventricular rate   63/min
- Atrial rhythm   Regular
- Atrial rate   63/min
- PRI: 0.20 second
- QRS: 0.06 second

RHYTHM IDENTIFICATION

Narrow-QRS tachycardia (supraventricular tachycardia [SVT]) with ST-segment depression
- Ventricular rhythm   Regular
- Ventricular rate   198/min
- Atrial rhythm   Unable to determine
- Atrial rate   Unable to determine
- PRI: Unable to determine
- QRS: 0.06 second

RHYTHM IDENTIFICATION

Second-degree AV block type I with multiformed PVCs and inverted T waves
- Ventricular rhythm   Irregular
- Ventricular rate   36 to 71/min
- Atrial rhythm   Regular except for the event(s)
- Atrial rate   79/min
- PRI: Lengthens
- QRS: 0.08 second

RHYTHM IDENTIFICATION

Junctional escape rhythm
- Ventricular rhythm   Regular
- Ventricular rate   44/min
- Atrial rhythm   Regular
- Atrial rate   44/min
- PRI: 0.12 second
- QRS: 0.06 second

RHYTHM IDENTIFICATION

Atrial fibrillation (uncontrolled)
- Ventricular rhythm   Irregular
- Ventricular rate   115 to 167/min
- Atrial rhythm   Unable to determine
- Atrial rate   Unable to determine
- PRI: Unable to determine
- QRS: 0.08 second

RHYTHM IDENTIFICATION

Sinus tachycardia
- Ventricular rhythm   Regular
- Ventricular rate   157/min
- Atrial rhythm   Regular
- Atrial rate   157/min
- PRI: 0.14 second
- QRS: 0.08 second

RHYTHM IDENTIFICATION

Sinus tachycardia with a run of ventricular tachycardia
- Ventricular rhythm   Regular except for the event
- Ventricular rate   135/min
- Atrial rhythm   Regular except for the event
- Atrial rate   135/min
- PRI: 0.12 second
- QRS: 0.08 to 0.10 second

◆ Identify the rhythm (lead II).

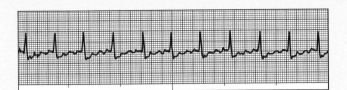

◆ Identify the rhythm (lead II).

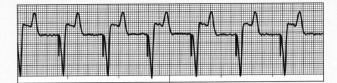

◆ This rhythm strip is from a 70-year-old woman with COPD. Identify the rhythm (lead II).

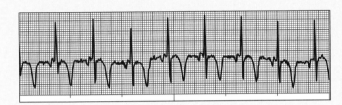

◆ This rhythm strip is from a 59-year-old woman complaining of dizziness. Blood pressure is 129/53. Blood sugar is 149. Identify the rhythm (lead II).

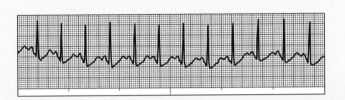

◆ Identify the rhythm (lead II).

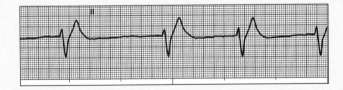

◆ This rhythm strip is from a 62-year-old diabetic with an altered level of responsiveness. Identify the rhythm (lead II).

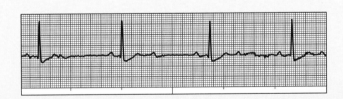

◆ This rhythm strip is from a 59-year-old man complaining of poor circulation in his legs. Blood pressure 106/68. Blood glucose is 95. Identify the rhythm (lead II).

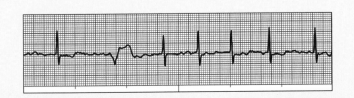

◆ Identify the rhythm (lead II).

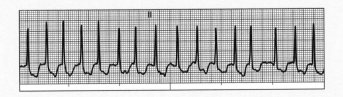

RHYTHM IDENTIFICATION

100% ventricular paced rhythm
- ◆ Atrial paced activity?   No
- ◆ Ventricular paced activity?   Yes
- ◆ Paced interval rate?   68

RHYTHM IDENTIFICATION

Atrial flutter
- ◆ Ventricular rhythm   Regular
- ◆ Ventricular rate   111/min
- ◆ Atrial rhythm   Unable to determine
- ◆ Atrial rate   Unable to determine
- ◆ PRI: Unable to determine
- ◆ QRS: 0.08 to 0.10 second

RHYTHM IDENTIFICATION

Sinus tachycardia
- ◆ Ventricular rhythm   Regular
- ◆ Ventricular rate   125/min
- ◆ Atrial rhythm   Regular
- ◆ Atrial rate   125/min
- ◆ PRI: 0.16 second
- ◆ QRS: 0.08 second

RHYTHM IDENTIFICATION

Accelerated junctional rhythm with inverted T waves
- ◆ Ventricular rhythm   Regular
- ◆ Ventricular rate   82/min
- ◆ Atrial rhythm   Regular
- ◆ Atrial rate   82/min
- ◆ PRI: 0.12 second
- ◆ QRS: 0.08 second

RHYTHM IDENTIFICATION

Second-degree AV block, 2:1 conduction, probably type I
- ◆ Ventricular rhythm   Regular
- ◆ Ventricular rate   35/min
- ◆ Atrial rhythm   Regular
- ◆ Atrial rate   70/min
- ◆ PRI: 0.28 second
- ◆ QRS: 0.06 second

RHYTHM IDENTIFICATION

Idioventricular (ventricular escape) rhythm
- ◆ Ventricular rhythm   Irregular
- ◆ Ventricular rate   30 to 41/min
- ◆ Atrial rhythm   Unable to determine
- ◆ Atrial rate   Unable to determine
- ◆ PRI: Unable to determine
- ◆ QRS: 0.16 second

RHYTHM IDENTIFICATION

Atrial fibrillation (uncontrolled) with ST-segment depression
- ◆ Ventricular rhythm   Irregular
- ◆ Ventricular rate   125 to 158/min
- ◆ Atrial rhythm   Unable to determine
- ◆ Atrial rate   Unable to determine
- ◆ PRI: Unable to determine
- ◆ QRS: 0.06 second

RHYTHM IDENTIFICATION

Atrial fibrillation with a ventricular complex
- ◆ Ventricular rhythm   Irregular
- ◆ Ventricular rate   68 to 88/min (atrial beats)
- ◆ Atrial rhythm   Unable to determine
- ◆ Atrial rate   Unable to determine
- ◆ PRI: Unable to determine
- ◆ QRS: 0.08 second (atrial beats)

RHYTHM IDENTIFICATION

- This rhythm strip is from a 61-year-old woman complaining of chest pain. She has a history of asthma and chronic obstructive pulmonary disease. Identify the rhythm.

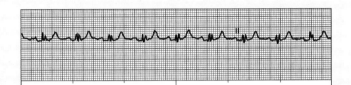

RHYTHM IDENTIFICATION

- This rhythm strip is from a 62-year-old woman complaining of chest pain. She has a history of 3 previous MIs and had a 3-vessel coronary artery bypass graft 10 years ago. Identify the rhythm (lead II).

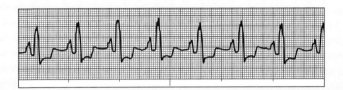

RHYTHM IDENTIFICATION

- Identify the rhythm (lead II).

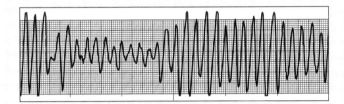

RHYTHM IDENTIFICATION

- Identify the rhythm (lead II).

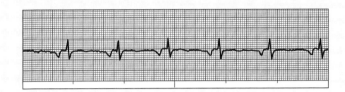

RHYTHM IDENTIFICATION

- This rhythm strip is from an asymptomatic 56-year-old man. Identify the rhythm (lead II).

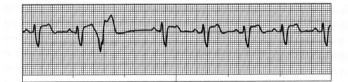

RHYTHM IDENTIFICATION

- This rhythm strip is from a 50-year-old man complaining of chest pain. Identify the rhythm (lead II).

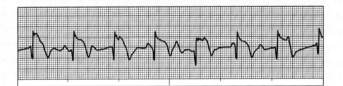

RHYTHM IDENTIFICATION

- Identify the rhythm (lead II).

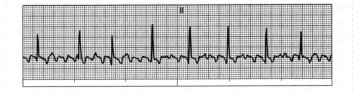

RHYTHM IDENTIFICATION

- This rhythm strip is from a 26-year-old man complaining of left flank pain. Identify the rhythm (lead II).

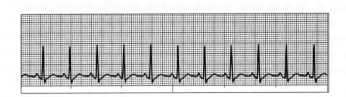

Sinus rhythm with a possible bundle branch block, notched P waves, ST-segment depression

- ◆ Ventricular rhythm   Regular
- ◆ Ventricular rate   75/min
- ◆ Atrial rhythm   Regular
- ◆ Atrial rate   75/min
- ◆ PRI: 0.16 second
- ◆ QRS: 0.10 to 0.12 second

Sinus rhythm (with a probable bundle branch block)

- ◆ Ventricular rhythm   Regular
- ◆ Ventricular rate   88/min
- ◆ Atrial rhythm   Regular
- ◆ Atrial rate   88/min
- ◆ PRI: 0.20 second
- ◆ QRS: 0.12 second

Accelerated junctional rhythm

- ◆ Ventricular rhythm   Regular
- ◆ Ventricular rate   62/min
- ◆ Atrial rhythm   Regular
- ◆ Atrial rate   62/min
- ◆ PRI: 0.14 second
- ◆ QRS: 0.08 second

Polymorphic ventricular tachycardia

- ◆ Ventricular rhythm   Irregular
- ◆ Ventricular rate   300 to 375/min
- ◆ Atrial rhythm   Unable to determine
- ◆ Atrial rate   Unable to determine
- ◆ PRI: Unable to determine
- ◆ QRS: Varies

Complete (third-degree) AV block with ST-segment elevation

- ◆ Ventricular rhythm   Regular
- ◆ Ventricular rate   75/min
- ◆ Atrial rhythm   Regular
- ◆ Atrial rate   107/min
- ◆ PRI: Varies
- ◆ QRS: 0.06 second

Sinus rhythm with a wide-QRS, R-on-T PVC, and ST-segment elevation

- ◆ Ventricular rhythm   Regular except for the event
- ◆ Ventricular rate   79/min (sinus beats)
- ◆ Atrial rhythm   Regular except for the event
- ◆ Atrial rate   79/min (sinus beats)
- ◆ PRI: 0.16 to 0.18 second (sinus beats)
- ◆ QRS: 0.12 second (sinus beats)

Sinus tachycardia

- ◆ Ventricular rhythm   Regular
- ◆ Ventricular rate   115/min
- ◆ Atrial rhythm   Regular
- ◆ Atrial rate   115/min
- ◆ PRI: 0.14 second
- ◆ QRS: 0.08 second

Atrial flutter

- ◆ Ventricular rhythm   Irregular
- ◆ Ventricular rate   70 to 100/min
- ◆ Atrial rhythm   Unable to determine
- ◆ Atrial rate   Unable to determine
- ◆ PRI: Unable to determine
- ◆ QRS: 0.08 second

RHYTHM IDENTIFICATION

◆ Identify the rhythm (lead II).

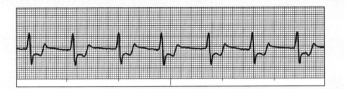

RHYTHM IDENTIFICATION

◆ This rhythm strip is from a 67-year-old woman complaining of dizziness and a "funny feeling" in her chest. She denies chest pain and is not short of breath. Identify the rhythm (lead II).

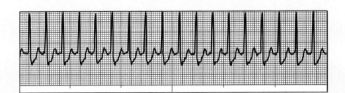

RHYTHM IDENTIFICATION

◆ Identify the rhythm (lead II).

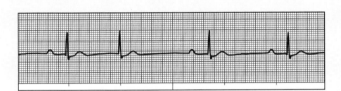

RHYTHM IDENTIFICATION

◆ This rhythm strip is from a 52-year-old woman found unresponsive, apneic, and pulseless. Identify the rhythm (lead II).

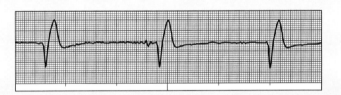

RHYTHM IDENTIFICATION

◆ Identify the rhythm (lead II).

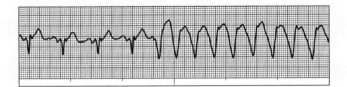

RHYTHM IDENTIFICATION

◆ Identify the rhythm (lead II).

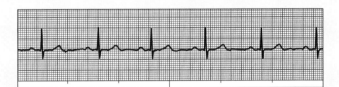

RHYTHM IDENTIFICATION

◆ Identify the rhythm (lead III).

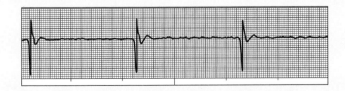

RHYTHM IDENTIFICATION

◆ This rhythm strip is from a 76-year-old man with an altered level of responsiveness. His blood pressure is 180/90. Blood sugar is 32. His skin is cool and dry. Identify the rhythm (lead II).

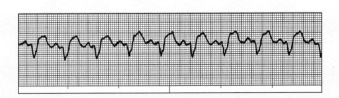

RHYTHM IDENTIFICATION

Narrow-QRS tachycardia (supraventricular tachycardia [SVT]) with ST-segment depression
- Ventricular rhythm   Regular
- Ventricular rate   186/min
- Atrial rhythm   Unable to determine
- Atrial rate   Unable to determine
- PRI: Unable to determine
- QRS: 0.06 second

RHYTHM IDENTIFICATION

Accelerated idioventricular rhythm (AIVR) with ST-segment depression
- Ventricular rhythm   Regular
- Ventricular rate   70/min
- Atrial rhythm   None
- Atrial rate   None
- PRI: None
- QRS: 0.12 second

RHYTHM IDENTIFICATION

Idioventricular (ventricular escape) rhythm
- Ventricular rhythm   Regular
- Ventricular rate   29/min
- Atrial rhythm   Unable to determine
- Atrial rate   Unable to determine
- PRI: Unable to determine
- QRS: 0.12 second

RHYTHM IDENTIFICATION

Sinus bradycardia with first-degree AV block and a PJC
- Ventricular rhythm   Regular except for the event
- Ventricular rate   40/min (sinus beats)
- Atrial rhythm   Regular except for the event
- Atrial rate   40/min (sinus beats)
- PRI: 0.36 second (sinus beats)
- QRS: 0.06 second (sinus beats)

RHYTHM IDENTIFICATION

Sinus bradycardia with first-degree AV block
- Ventricular rhythm   Regular
- Ventricular rate   56/min
- Atrial rhythm   Regular
- Atrial rate   56/min
- PRI: 0.24 second
- QRS: 0.06 to 0.08 second

RHYTHM IDENTIFICATION

Sinus rhythm to monomorphic ventricular tachycardia (VT)
- Ventricular rhythm   Regular (sinus beats), regular (VT)
- Ventricular rate   94/min (sinus beats) to 150/min (VT)
- Atrial rhythm   Regular to unable to determine
- Atrial rate   94/min (sinus beats)
- PRI: 0.16 second (sinus beats)
- QRS: 0.10 second (sinus beats) to 0.14 second (VT)

RHYTHM IDENTIFICATION

Sinus rhythm with a wide-QRS and ST-segment elevation
- Ventricular rhythm   Regular
- Ventricular rate   94/min
- Atrial rhythm   Regular
- Atrial rate   94/min
- PRI: 0.20 second
- QRS: 0.12 second

RHYTHM IDENTIFICATION

Atrial fibrillation
- Ventricular rhythm   Regular
- Ventricular rate   29/min
- Atrial rhythm   Unable to determine
- Atrial rate   Unable to determine
- PRI: Unable to determine
- QRS: 0.10 second

Note: This patient was diagnosed with digitalis toxicity.

◆ Identify the rhythm (lead II).

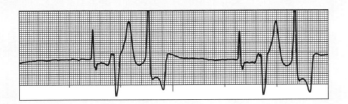

◆ Identify the rhythm (lead II).

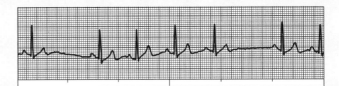

◆ Identify the rhythm (lead II).

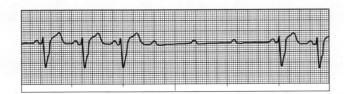

◆ This rhythm strip is from a 36-year-old woman last seen 4 hours ago. She is unresponsive, apneic, and pulseless. She has a history of congestive heart failure and depression. Identify the rhythm.

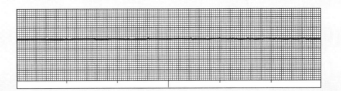

◆ This rhythm strip is from a 67-year-old woman complaining of chest pain. Identify the rhythm (lead II).

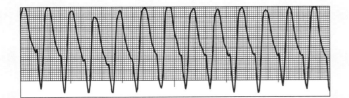

◆ Identify the rhythm.

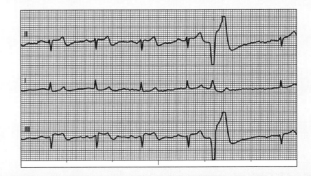

◆ Identify the rhythm.

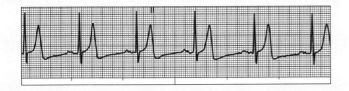

◆ Identify the rhythm (lead II).

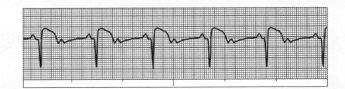

RHYTHM IDENTIFICATION

Sinus rhythm with nonconducted PACs
- Ventricular rhythm   Regular except for the event
- Ventricular rate   79/min
- Atrial rhythm   Regular except for the event
- Atrial rate   79/min
- PRI: 0.16 second
- QRS: 0.06 second

RHYTHM IDENTIFICATION

Junctional bradycardia with multiform PVCs
- Ventricular rhythm   Irregular
- Ventricular rate   21 to 25/min (junctional beats)
- Atrial rhythm   None
- Atrial rate   None
- PRI: None
- QRS: 0.06 to 0.08 second (junctional beats)

RHYTHM IDENTIFICATION

Asystole
- Ventricular rhythm   None
- Ventricular rate   None
- Atrial rhythm   None
- Atrial rate   None
- PRI: None
- QRS: None

RHYTHM IDENTIFICATION

Second-degree AV block type II
- Ventricular rhythm   Irregular
- Ventricular rate   20 to 79/min
- Atrial rhythm   Regular
- Atrial rate   79/min
- PRI: 0.14 second
- QRS: 0.16 second

RHYTHM IDENTIFICATION

Sinus rhythm with first-degree AV block and a PVC
- Ventricular rhythm   Regular except for the PVC
- Ventricular rate   63/min (sinus beats)
- Atrial rhythm   Regular except for the PVC
- Atrial rate   63/min (sinus beats)
- PRI: 0.24 second
- QRS: 0.08 second

RHYTHM IDENTIFICATION

Monomorphic ventricular tachycardia
- Ventricular rhythm   Regular
- Ventricular rate   125/min
- Atrial rhythm   Unable to determine
- Atrial rate   Unable to determine
- PRI: Unable to determine
- QRS: 0.16 to 0.18 second

RHYTHM IDENTIFICATION

Second-degree AV block, 2:1 conduction, probably type I with ST-segment elevation
- Ventricular rhythm   Regular
- Ventricular rate   55/min
- Atrial rhythm   Regular
- Atrial rate   107/min
- PRI: 0.16 second
- QRS: 0.06 second

RHYTHM IDENTIFICATION

Sinus bradycardia with tall T waves
- Ventricular rhythm   Regular
- Ventricular rate   55/min
- Atrial rhythm   Regular
- Atrial rate   55/min
- PRI: 0.20 second
- QRS: 0.08 second

RHYTHM IDENTIFICATION

◆ Identify the rhythm (lead II).

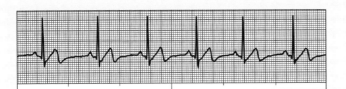

RHYTHM IDENTIFICATION

◆ Identify the rhythm (lead II).

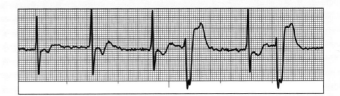

RHYTHM IDENTIFICATION

◆ Identify the rhythm.

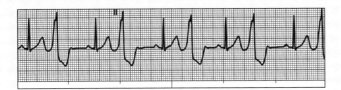

RHYTHM IDENTIFICATION

◆ Identify the rhythm (lead II).

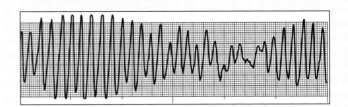

RHYTHM IDENTIFICATION

◆ Identify the rhythm (lead II).

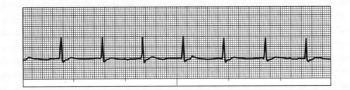

RHYTHM IDENTIFICATION

◆ Identify the rhythm (lead II).

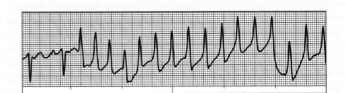

RHYTHM IDENTIFICATION

◆ Identify the rhythm.

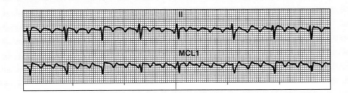

RHYTHM IDENTIFICATION

◆ Identify the rhythm (lead II).

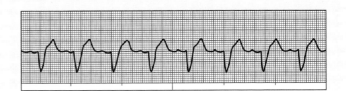

RHYTHM IDENTIFICATION

Atrial fibrillation with uniform PVCs, inverted T waves
- ◆ Ventricular rhythm   Irregular
- ◆ Ventricular rate   32 to 75/min (atrial beats)
- ◆ Atrial rhythm   Unable to determine
- ◆ Atrial rate   Unable to determine
- ◆ PRI: Unable to determine
- ◆ QRS: 0.10 second (atrial beats)

RHYTHM IDENTIFICATION

Sinus arrhythmia
- ◆ Ventricular rhythm   Irregular
- ◆ Ventricular rate   54 to 65/min
- ◆ Atrial rhythm   Irregular
- ◆ Atrial rate   54 to 65/min
- ◆ PRI: 0.18 second
- ◆ QRS: 0.08 second

RHYTHM IDENTIFICATION

Polymorphic ventricular tachycardia
- ◆ Ventricular rhythm   Irregular
- ◆ Ventricular rate   300 to 375/min
- ◆ Atrial rhythm   Unable to determine
- ◆ Atrial rate   Unable to determine
- ◆ PRI: Unable to determine
- ◆ QRS: Varies

RHYTHM IDENTIFICATION

Sinus bradycardia with ventricular bigeminy
- ◆ Ventricular rhythm   Regular except for the event (every other beat is an ectopic beat)
- ◆ Ventricular rate   45/min (sinus beats)
- ◆ Atrial rhythm   Regular except for the event
- ◆ Atrial rate   45/min (sinus beats)
- ◆ PRI: 0.18 second (sinus beats)
- ◆ QRS: 0.06 second (sinus beats)

RHYTHM IDENTIFICATION

Sinus rhythm to narrow-QRS tachycardia
- ◆ Ventricular rhythm   Irregular
- ◆ Ventricular rate   91 to 188/min
- ◆ Atrial rhythm   Irregular
- ◆ Atrial rate   91/min to unable to determine
- ◆ PRI: 0.18 second to unable to determine
- ◆ QRS: 0.10 (sinus beats) to 0.08 to 0.11 second

RHYTHM IDENTIFICATION

Accelerated junctional rhythm
- ◆ Ventricular rhythm   Regular
- ◆ Ventricular rate   76/min
- ◆ Atrial rhythm   None
- ◆ Atrial rate   None
- ◆ PRI: None
- ◆ QRS: 0.06 second

RHYTHM IDENTIFICATION

Sinus rhythm with a wide-QRS and ST-segment elevation
- ◆ Ventricular rhythm   Regular
- ◆ Ventricular rate   83/min
- ◆ Atrial rhythm   Regular
- ◆ Atrial rate   83/min
- ◆ PRI: 0.20 second
- ◆ QRS: 0.12 second

RHYTHM IDENTIFICATION

Atrial flutter
- ◆ Ventricular rhythm   Irregular
- ◆ Ventricular rate   58 to 79/min
- ◆ Atrial rhythm   Unable to determine
- ◆ Atrial rate   Unable to determine
- ◆ PRI: Unable to determine
- ◆ QRS: 0.10 second

RHYTHM IDENTIFICATION

◆ Identify the rhythm (lead II).

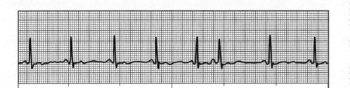

RHYTHM IDENTIFICATION

◆ Identify the rhythm (lead II).

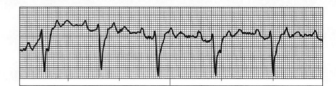

RHYTHM IDENTIFICATION

◆ Identify the rhythm (lead II).

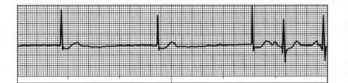

RHYTHM IDENTIFICATION

◆ Identify the rhythm (lead II).

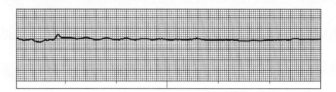

RHYTHM IDENTIFICATION

◆ This rhythm strip is from a 71-year-old woman with vomitus that looks like coffee grounds. She has a history of esophageal cancer. Blood pressure is 130/60. Identify the rhythm (lead II).

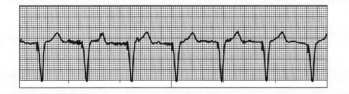

RHYTHM IDENTIFICATION

◆ Identify the rhythm.

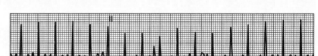

RHYTHM IDENTIFICATION

◆ Identify the rhythm (lead III).

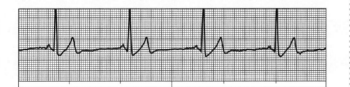

RHYTHM IDENTIFICATION

◆ Identify the rhythm (lead II).

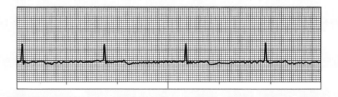

RHYTHM IDENTIFICATION

Second-degree AV block, 2:1 conduction, probably type 2 with ST-segment depression

- ◆ Ventricular rhythm   Regular
- ◆ Ventricular rate   54/min
- ◆ Atrial rhythm   Regular
- ◆ Atrial rate   107/min
- ◆ PRI: 0.28 second
- ◆ QRS: 0.16 to 0.20 second

RHYTHM IDENTIFICATION

Sinus rhythm with a PAC

- ◆ Ventricular rhythm   Regular except for the event
- ◆ Ventricular rate   71/min
- ◆ Atrial rhythm   Regular except for the event
- ◆ Atrial rate   71/min
- ◆ PRI: 0.12 second
- ◆ QRS: 0.06 second

RHYTHM IDENTIFICATION

Fine ventricular fibrillation to asystole

- ◆ Ventricular rhythm   Unable to determine
- ◆ Ventricular rate   Unable to determine
- ◆ Atrial rhythm   Unable to determine
- ◆ Atrial rate   Unable to determine
- ◆ PRI: Unable to determine
- ◆ QRS: Unable to determine

RHYTHM IDENTIFICATION

Junctional bradycardia to sinus rhythm

- ◆ Ventricular rhythm   Regular (junctional beats); unable to determine (sinus beats)
- ◆ Ventricular rate   30/min (junctional beats); unable to determine (sinus beats)
- ◆ Atrial rhythm   None (junctional beats); unable to determine (sinus beats)
- ◆ Atrial rate   None (junctional beats) to 75/min (sinus beats)
- ◆ PRI: None (junctional beats) to 0.18 (sinus beats)
- ◆ QRS: 0.04 second (junctional beats) to 0.08 second (sinus beats)

RHYTHM IDENTIFICATION

Sinus tachycardia

- ◆ Ventricular rhythm   Regular
- ◆ Ventricular rate   167/min
- ◆ Atrial rhythm   Regular
- ◆ Atrial rate   167/min
- ◆ PRI: 0.12 second
- ◆ QRS: 0.06 second

RHYTHM IDENTIFICATION

100% ventricular paced rhythm

- ◆ Atrial paced activity?   No
- ◆ Ventricular paced activity?   Yes
- ◆ Paced interval rate?   72

RHYTHM IDENTIFICATION

Atrial fibrillation

- ◆ Ventricular rhythm   Regular
- ◆ Ventricular rate   39/min
- ◆ Atrial rhythm   Unable to determine
- ◆ Atrial rate   Unable to determine
- ◆ PRI: Unable to determine
- ◆ QRS: 0.04 to 0.06 second

Note: This patient was diagnosed with digitalis toxicity.

RHYTHM IDENTIFICATION

Sinus bradycardia with ST-segment depression

- ◆ Ventricular rhythm   Regular
- ◆ Ventricular rate   46/min
- ◆ Atrial rhythm   Regular
- ◆ Atrial rate   46/min
- ◆ PRI: 0.14 second
- ◆ QRS: 0.10 second

RHYTHM IDENTIFICATION

◆ This rhythm strip is from an 89-year-old man with an altered level of responsiveness. Identify the rhythm (lead II).

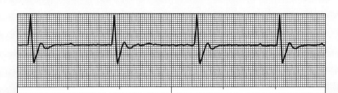

RHYTHM IDENTIFICATION

◆ Identify the rhythm (lead II).

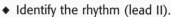
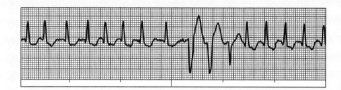

RHYTHM IDENTIFICATION

◆ This rhythm strip is from a 51-year-old man found unresponsive. He has a history of esophageal varices and gastrointestinal bleeding. Blood pressure is 182/100. Identify the rhythm (lead I).

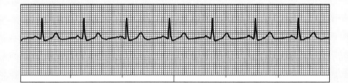

RHYTHM IDENTIFICATION

◆ This rhythm strip is from a 66-year-old woman complaining of abdominal pain and weakness that began suddenly while eating breakfast. Blood pressure is 102/62. Identify the rhythm (lead II).

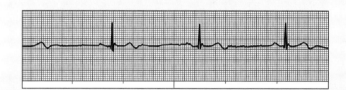

RHYTHM IDENTIFICATION

◆ This rhythm strip is from a 63-year-old man that collapsed on the kitchen floor. He is unresponsive, apneic, and without a pulse. His past medical history includes a coronary artery bypass graft 8 years ago and pacemaker implantation 5 years ago. Identify the rhythm (lead II).

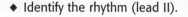
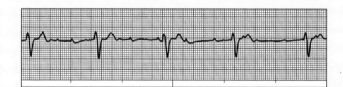

RHYTHM IDENTIFICATION

◆ Identify the rhythm (lead II).

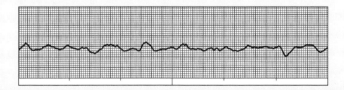

RHYTHM IDENTIFICATION

◆ Identify the rhythm (lead III).

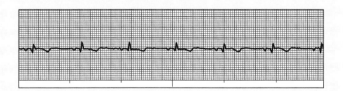

RHYTHM IDENTIFICATION

◆ Identify the rhythm (lead II).

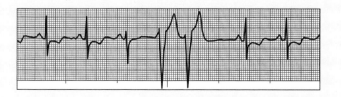

RHYTHM IDENTIFICATION

Atrial fibrillation with a run of ventricular complexes
- Ventricular rhythm — Irregular
- Ventricular rate — 143 to 167/min (atrial beats)
- Atrial rhythm — Unable to determine
- Atrial rate — Unable to determine
- PRI: — Unable to determine
- QRS: — 0.08 second (atrial beats)

RHYTHM IDENTIFICATION

Complete (third-degree) AV block with ST-segment depression
- Ventricular rhythm — Regular
- Ventricular rate — 38/min
- Atrial rhythm — Regular
- Atrial rate — 51/min
- PRI: — Varies
- QRS: — 0.16 second

RHYTHM IDENTIFICATION

Sinus bradycardia with first-degree AV block
- Ventricular rhythm — Regular
- Ventricular rate — 37/min
- Atrial rhythm — Regular
- Atrial rate — 37/min
- PRI: — 0.22 second
- QRS: — 0.06 to 0.08 second

RHYTHM IDENTIFICATION

Sinus rhythm
- Ventricular rhythm — Regular
- Ventricular rate — 75/min
- Atrial rhythm — Regular
- Atrial rate — 75/min
- PRI: — 0.12 second
- QRS: — 0.08 second

RHYTHM IDENTIFICATION

Complete (third-degree) AV block
- Ventricular rhythm — Regular
- Ventricular rate — 46/min
- Atrial rhythm — Regular
- Atrial rate — 107/min
- PRI: — Varies
- QRS: — 0.14 second

RHYTHM IDENTIFICATION

Ventricular fibrillation
- Ventricular rhythm — Unable to determine
- Ventricular rate — Unable to determine
- Atrial rhythm — Unable to determine
- Atrial rate — Unable to determine
- PRI: — Unable to determine
- QRS: — Unable to determine

RHYTHM IDENTIFICATION

Sinus rhythm with a pair of PVCs, ST-segment depression, and inverted T waves
- Ventricular rhythm — Regular except for the event(s)
- Ventricular rate — 79/min (sinus beats)
- Atrial rhythm — Regular except for the event(s)
- Atrial rate — 79/min (sinus beats)
- PRI: — 0.16 second (sinus beats)
- QRS: — 0.06 to 0.08 second (sinus beats)

RHYTHM IDENTIFICATION

Accelerated junctional rhythm
- Ventricular rhythm — Regular
- Ventricular rate — 65/min
- Atrial rhythm — Regular
- Atrial rate — 65/min
- PRI: — 0.18 second
- QRS: — 0.08 second

RHYTHM IDENTIFICATION

◆ Identify the rhythm (lead II).

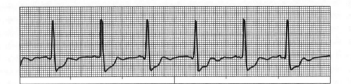

RHYTHM IDENTIFICATION

◆ Identify the rhythm (lead II).

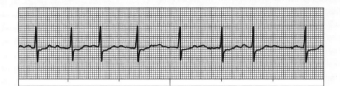

RHYTHM IDENTIFICATION

◆ Identify the rhythm (lead II).

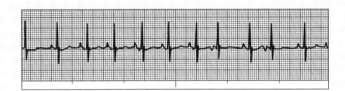

RHYTHM IDENTIFICATION

◆ This rhythm strip is from a 61-year-old man found unresponsive, apneic, and pulseless. Identify the rhythm (lead II).

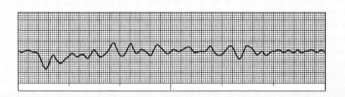

RHYTHM IDENTIFICATION

◆ This rhythm strip is from a 20-year-old woman who collapsed on the sidewalk of her residence. A family member states she has a history of supraventricular tachycardia and takes atenolol. Blood pressure is 102/42.

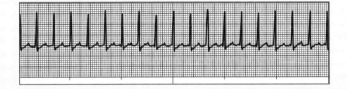

RHYTHM IDENTIFICATION

◆ This rhythm strip is from a 27-year-old man with a stab wound to his mid-abdomen. Blood pressure is 126/68. Identify the rhythm.

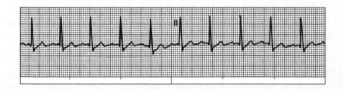

RHYTHM IDENTIFICATION

◆ Identify the rhythm (lead II).

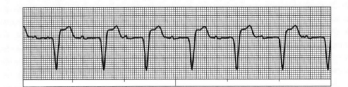

RHYTHM IDENTIFICATION

◆ This rhythm strip is from an 82-year-old man complaining of chest pain and difficulty breathing. Identify the rhythm (lead II).

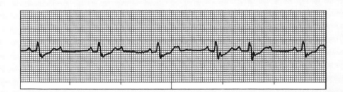

RHYTHM IDENTIFICATION

Atrial fibrillation (controlled)
- ◆ Ventricular rhythm   Irregular
- ◆ Ventricular rate   71 to 107/min
- ◆ Atrial rhythm   Unable to determine
- ◆ Atrial rate   Unable to determine
- ◆ PRI: Unable to determine
- ◆ QRS: 0.08 second

RHYTHM IDENTIFICATION

Sinus rhythm with ST-segment depression
- ◆ Ventricular rhythm   Regular
- ◆ Ventricular rate   65/min
- ◆ Atrial rhythm   Regular
- ◆ Atrial rate   65/min
- ◆ PRI: 0.16 second
- ◆ QRS: 0.08 second

RHYTHM IDENTIFICATION

Ventricular fibrillation (VF) (changing from coarse to fine VF)
- ◆ Ventricular rhythm   Unable to determine
- ◆ Ventricular rate   Unable to determine
- ◆ Atrial rhythm   Unable to determine
- ◆ Atrial rate   Unable to determine
- ◆ PRI: Unable to determine
- ◆ QRS: Unable to determine

RHYTHM IDENTIFICATION

Sinus tachycardia with PJCs
- ◆ Ventricular rhythm   Regular except for the event(s)
- ◆ Ventricular rate   111/min
- ◆ Atrial rhythm   Regular except for the event(s)
- ◆ Atrial rate   111/min
- ◆ PRI: 0.12 second (sinus beats)
- ◆ QRS: 0.06 second

RHYTHM IDENTIFICATION

Sinus rhythm
- ◆ Ventricular rhythm   Regular
- ◆ Ventricular rate   98/min
- ◆ Atrial rhythm   Regular
- ◆ Atrial rate   98/min
- ◆ PRI: 0.16 second
- ◆ QRS: 0.08 second

RHYTHM IDENTIFICATION

Narrow-QRS tachycardia (supraventricular tachycardia [SVT])
- ◆ Ventricular rhythm   Regular
- ◆ Ventricular rate   188/min
- ◆ Atrial rhythm   Unable to determine
- ◆ Atrial rate   Unable to determine
- ◆ PRI: Unable to determine
- ◆ QRS: 0.06 second

RHYTHM IDENTIFICATION

Second-degree AV block type I (with short period of 2:1 conduction), ST-segment depression
- ◆ Ventricular rhythm   Irregular
- ◆ Ventricular rate   52 to 94/min
- ◆ Atrial rhythm   Regular
- ◆ Atrial rate   100/min
- ◆ PRI: Lengthens
- ◆ QRS: 0.08 second

RHYTHM IDENTIFICATION

Sinus rhythm with first-degree AV block, ST-segment elevation
- ◆ Ventricular rhythm   Regular
- ◆ Ventricular rate   75/min
- ◆ Atrial rhythm   Regular
- ◆ Atrial rate   75/min
- ◆ PRI: 0.36 second
- ◆ QRS: 0.10 to 0.11 second

RHYTHM IDENTIFICATION

- ◆ This rhythm strip is from a 63-year-old woman complaining of palpitations. Identify the rhythm (lead II).

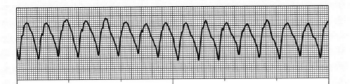

RHYTHM IDENTIFICATION

- ◆ Identify the rhythm (lead II).

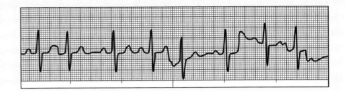

RHYTHM IDENTIFICATION

- ◆ Identify the rhythm (lead II).

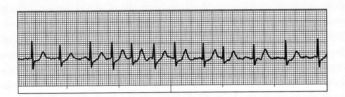

RHYTHM IDENTIFICATION

- ◆ This rhythm strip is from a 54-year-old woman found unresponsive, apneic, and pulseless. Her past medical history includes diabetes and a MI 5 years ago. Identify the rhythm (lead II).

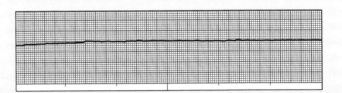

RHYTHM IDENTIFICATION

- ◆ Identify the rhythm (lead II).

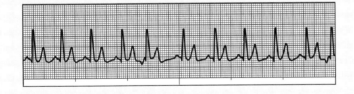

RHYTHM IDENTIFICATION

- ◆ Identify the rhythm (lead II).

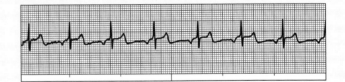

RHYTHM IDENTIFICATION

- ◆ This rhythm strip is from a 57-year-old man that stepped out of the bed of his pickup truck and fell head first into a shed. His present complaint is neck pain. Blood pressure is 110/78. Identify the rhythm (lead II).

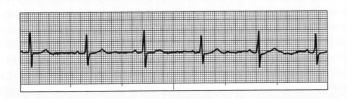

RHYTHM IDENTIFICATION

- ◆ Identify the rhythm (lead II).

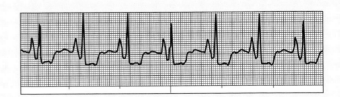

Sinus rhythm with a wide-QRS and PACs
- Ventricular rhythm   Regular except for the event(s)
- Ventricular rate   79/min (sinus beats)
- Atrial rhythm   Regular except for the event(s)
- Atrial rate   79/min (sinus beats)
- PRI: 0.20 second (sinus beats)
- QRS: 0.12 second (sinus beats)

Monomorphic ventricular tachycardia
- Ventricular rhythm   Regular
- Ventricular rate   150/min
- Atrial rhythm   Unable to determine
- Atrial rate   Unable to determine
- PRI: Unable to determine
- QRS: 0.14 second

Asystole
- Ventricular rhythm   None
- Ventricular rate   None
- Atrial rhythm   None
- Atrial rate   None
- PRI: None
- QRS: None

Atrial fibrillation (uncontrolled)
- Ventricular rhythm   Irregular
- Ventricular rate   100 to 167/min
- Atrial rhythm   Unable to determine
- Atrial rate   Unable to determine
- PRI: Unable to determine
- QRS: 0.08 second

Accelerated junctional rhythm
- Ventricular rhythm   Regular
- Ventricular rate   79/min
- Atrial rhythm   Regular
- Atrial rate   79/min
- PRI: 0.10 second
- QRS: 0.08 second

Sinus tachycardia with PJCs
- Ventricular rhythm   Regular except for the event(s)
- Ventricular rate   107/min
- Atrial rhythm   Regular except for the event(s)
- Atrial rate   107/min
- PRI: 0.14 second (sinus beats)
- QRS: 0.08 second

Sinus rhythm with ST-segment depression and inverted T waves
- Ventricular rhythm   Regular
- Ventricular rate   67/min
- Atrial rhythm   Regular
- Atrial rate   67/min
- PRI: 0.16 second
- QRS: 0.08 second

Sinus bradycardia
- Ventricular rhythm   Regular
- Ventricular rate   55/min
- Atrial rhythm   Regular
- Atrial rate   55/min
- PRI: 0.20 second
- QRS: 0.08 second

◆ This rhythm strip is from a 90-year-old unresponsive woman. She has a history of congestive heart failure. Her medications include furosemide and albuterol. Identify the rhythm.

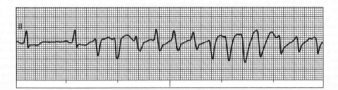

◆ Identify the rhythm.

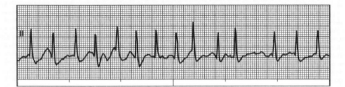

Sinus rhythm with ST-segment depression to polymorphic ventricular tachycardia

◆ Ventricular rhythm   Regular (sinus beats) to irregular (ventricular beats)
◆ Ventricular rate   65/min (sinus beats) to approximately 167 to 214 (ventricular beats)
◆ Atrial rhythm   Regular (sinus beats)
◆ Atrial rate   65/min (sinus beats)
◆ PRI: 0.16 second (sinus beats)
◆ QRS: 0.10 to 0.12 second (sinus beats)

Atrial fibrillation

◆ Ventricular rhythm   Irregular
◆ Ventricular rate   77 to 188/min
◆ Atrial rhythm   Unable to determine
◆ Atrial rate   Unable to determine
◆ PRI: Unable to determine
◆ QRS: 0.06 to 0.08 second

ILLUSTRATION CREDITS

Anatomy & Physiology Review

Aehlert B: *ACLS Quick Review Study Guide,* St. Louis, 1994, Mosby.

Crawford M, Spence M: *Commonsense Approach to Coronary Care,* ed 6, St. Louis, 1995, Mosby.

Goldberger A: *Clinical Electrocardiography: A Simplified Approach,* ed 6, St. Louis, 1999, Mosby.

Grauer K: *A Practical Guide to ECG Interpretation,* ed 2, St. Louis, 1998 Mosby.

Guyton A, Hall J: *Textbook of Medical Physiology,* ed 9, Philadelphia, 1996, W.B. Saunders.

Herlihy B, Maebius N: *The Human Body in Health and Illness,* Philadelphia, 2000, W. B. Saunders.

Sanders M: *Mosby's Paramedic Textbook,* ed 1, St. Louis, 1994, Mosby.

Thelan L, Urden L, Lough M, et al: *Critical Care Nursing: Diagnosis and Management,* ed 2, St. Louis, 1998, Mosby.

Thibodeau G, Patton K: *Anatomy and Physiology,* ed 4, St. Louis, 1999, Mosby.